Ocular Pathology
Case Reviews

Executive Content Strategist: Russell Gabbedy
Senior Content Development Specialist: Sharon Nash
Senior Project Manager: Beula Christopher
Design: Miles Hitchen
Marketing Manager(s) (UK/USA): Gaynor Jones/Kathleen Reid

Ocular Pathology
Case Reviews

Amir A. Azari, MD
Clinical Assistant Professor
Wills Eye Institute
Jefferson Medical College of Thomas Jefferson University
Philadelphia, PA, USA

Daniel M. Albert, MD, MS
F.A. Davis Professor, Department of Ophthalmology and Visual Sciences, University of
Wisconsin School of Medicine and Public Health
Founding Director, University of Wisconsin McPherson Eye Research Institute
Madison, WI, USA

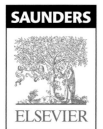

London, New York, Oxford, Philadelphia, St Louis, Sydney, Toronto 2015

ELSEVIER
SAUNDERS

ISBN: 978-0-323-28795-1
e-book ISBN: 978-0-323-28796-8
Printed in China
Last digit is the print number: 9   8   7   6   5   4   3   2   1

Contents

Preface

The goal of this book is to provide clinicians with the ability to look at images of the important lesions of the eye and adnexa so they can more quickly and accurately make the diagnosis. This facility is achieved by providing case studies with representative clinical pictures, accompanied by the histopathological appearance of that lesion. As residents and fellows, we gain experience in "sight recognition" of lesions as viewed directly on the lids and external surface of the eye or by slit-lamp, ophthalmoscope or an imaging study. Some lesions are sufficiently distinctive to be diagnosed based on "sight recognition" without analysis. Often, however, they suggest more than one possibility, i.e., a differential diagnosis. Analysis of both the clinical evidence and histopathology is necessary to make a final correct diagnosis.

This book highlights 200 frequently encountered or challenging examples of ocular and adnexal disorders, together with their associated pathologic appearance. It attempts to simulate what the clinician experiences when examining the patient in a clinical setting, by presenting each case initially as an "unknown", without specifically pointing out to the reader the diagnostic, clinical, and pathologic features that characterize the diagnosis. The reader must then analyze, on his or her own, the clinical or differential diagnosis, and then the confirming pathologic diagnosis. Supporting pages for each case present the same images accompanied by concise labels indicating the key points to be noted in order to make the correct diagnosis. This enables the reader to determine if his or her interpretation and diagnosis is accurate.

In this manner, utilizing self-instruction, *Ocular Pathology Case Reviews* enables ophthalmologists to recognize those features necessary to make correct diagnoses. With repetition, his or her ability to analyze, interpret, and make that diagnosis is reinforced, and the clinical appearance and histological features become correlated in a manner closely approximating that of clinical experience.

Clinicians who have a firm grasp of the clinical–pathologic correlation are better able to meet the challenges of everyday clinical practice, allowing for a high quality and more enjoyable experience that ultimately benefits patients. Whether used as an initial learning tool, or as a method of review, the authors believe *Ocular Pathology Case Reviews* will be an effective and enjoyable support to you in your practice of ophthalmology.

Amir A. Azari, MD
Daniel M. Albert, MD, MS

Acknowledgments

The authors express their gratitude to Drs Mozghan Rezai Kanavi and Heather Potter for their assistance and encouragement in compiling this book. Drs Neal Barney, Sarah Nehls, Jason Sokol, and Justin Gottlieb generously helped in providing clinical photographs. Laura Cruz and Patty Rasmussen provided valuable assistance in its preparation. Vicky Rogness has meticulously prepared the high quality slides that are used in this book. Russell Gabbedy, Executive Content Strategist, and Sharon Nash, Senior Content Development Specialist, of Elsevier guided this book through the editorial and publishing process with expertise, insight, and graciousness.

Dedication

This book is dedicated to
our wives for their love, patience, and support

Diagnosis: Basal cell carcinoma.

Clinical description: A raised telangiectatic lesion with associated madarosis is present in the left lower eyelid.

Histological description: Histopathology demonstrates tissue covered with keratinized stratified squamous epithelium. The dermis contains cords, and islands of basaloid cells, which exhibit peripheral palisading of their nuclei. A retraction artifact is seen.

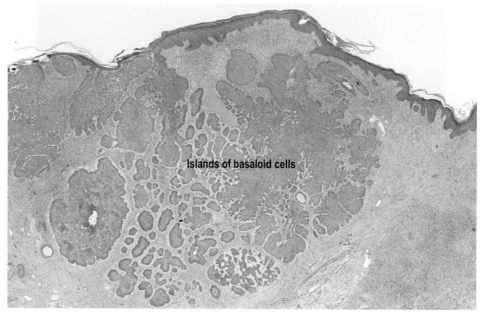

Islands of basaloid cells

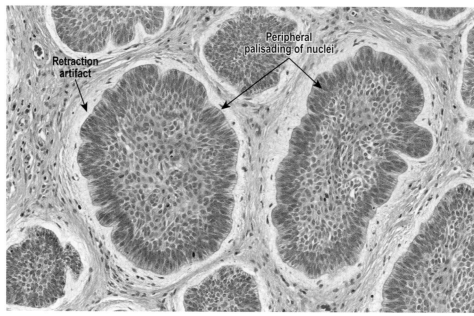

Peripheral palisading of nuclei

Retraction artifact

Dedication

This book is dedicated to
our wives for their love, patience, and support

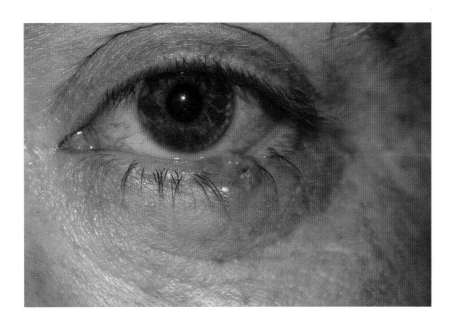

A 67-year-old woman presented with a left lower eyelid lesion. Excisional biopsy of the lesion demonstrates the histological findings shown below.

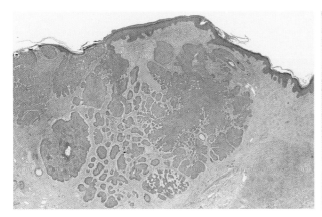

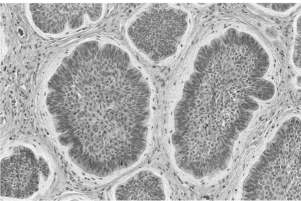

Diagnosis: Basal cell carcinoma.

Clinical description: A raised telangiectatic lesion with associated madarosis is present in the left lower eyelid.

Histological description: Histopathology demonstrates tissue covered with keratinized stratified squamous epithelium. The dermis contains cords, and islands of basaloid cells, which exhibit peripheral palisading of their nuclei. A retraction artifact is seen.

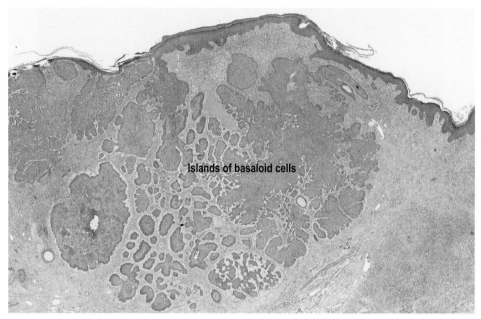

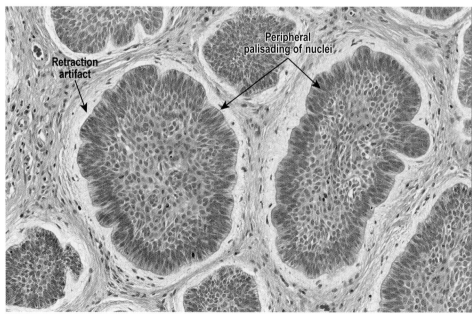

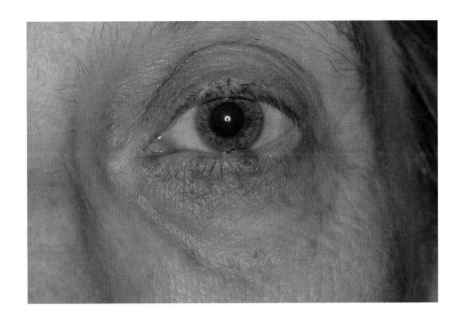

A 68-year-old woman presented with a red, itchy left lower eyelid lesion present for the past 3 months.

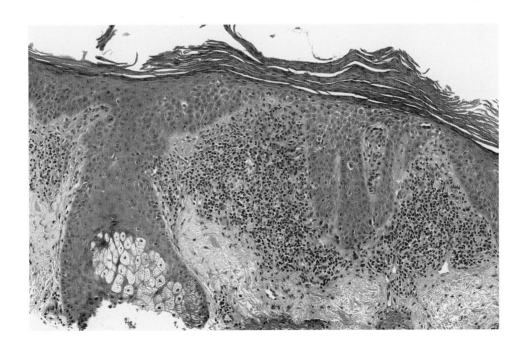

Diagnosis: Actinic keratosis.

Clinical description: A red, minimally elevated, scaly lesion at the margin of the left lower lid is demonstrated.

Histological description: Variable amounts of hyperkeratosis (increased thickness of the keratin layer), parakeratosis (presence of nuclei in the keratin layer), and acanthosis (thickening of the prickle cell layer) is seen. There is some atypia in the basal layer. Mild nongranulomatous inflammation is seen within the dermis.

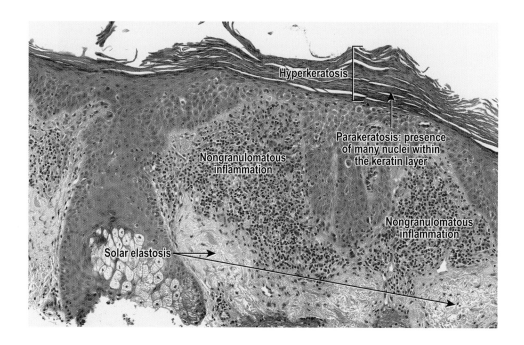

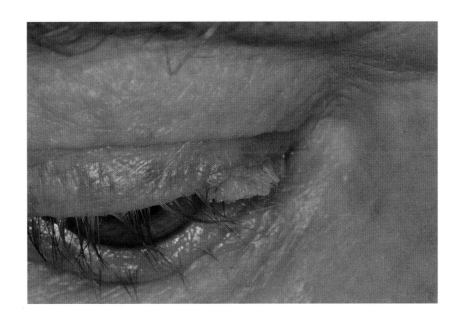

A 67-year-old woman presented with a 5-month history of a right eyelid lesion.

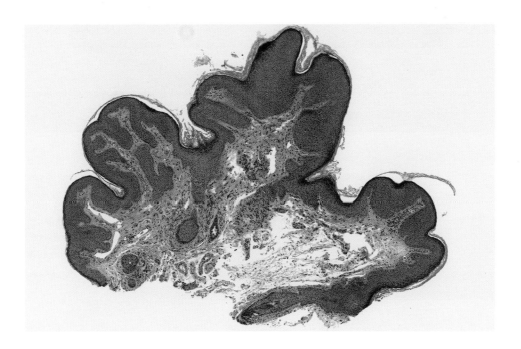

Diagnosis: Squamous cell papilloma.

Clinical description: Clinical examination reveals a partially keratinized papillomatous right upper eyelid lesion.

Histological description: Histopathology reveals a lesion covered by keratinized stratified squamous epithelium and exhibiting acanthosis and papillary projections.

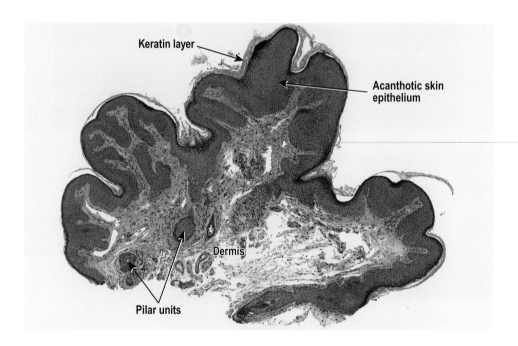

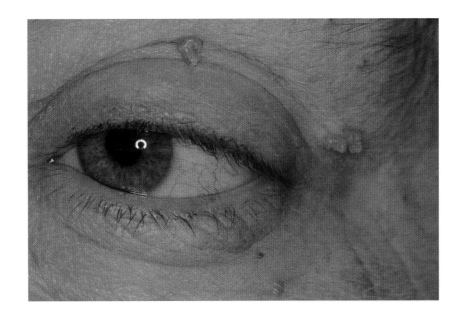

A 72-year-old woman presented with multiple eyelid lesions.

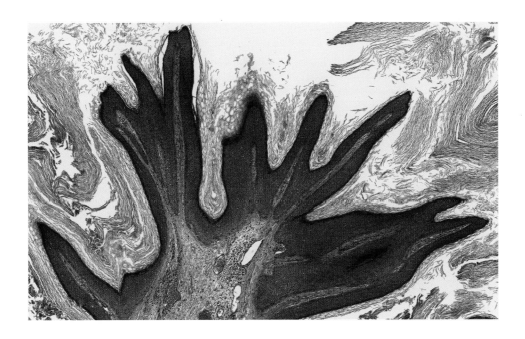

Diagnosis: Verruca vulgaris.

Clinical description: Clinical examination shows multiple keratinized lesions on the upper and lower eyelids.

Histological description: Histopathology reveals fronds of hyperkeratotic stratified squamous epithelium lining a fibrovascular dermis.

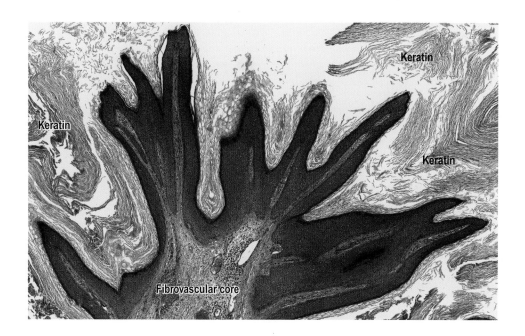

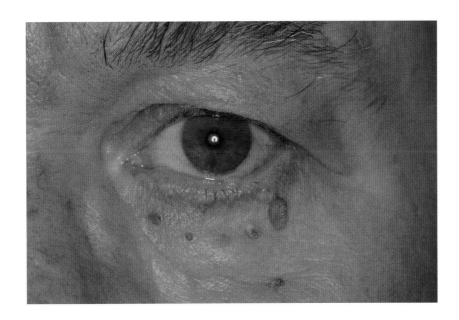

A 61-year-old man presented with multiple skin tags. The skin tags were removed in the doctor's office.

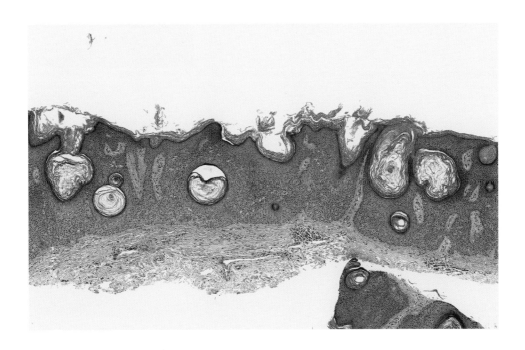

Diagnosis: Seborrheic keratosis (sessile).

Clinical description: Multiple pigmented lesions with a "stuck-on" appearance are seen.

Histological description: Histopathology reveals mildly acanthotic, keratinized, stratified squamous epithelium with pseudohorn cysts (asterisks).

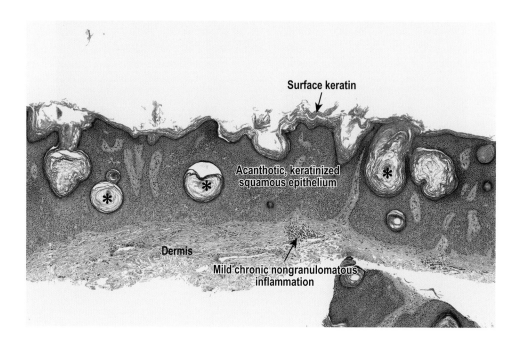

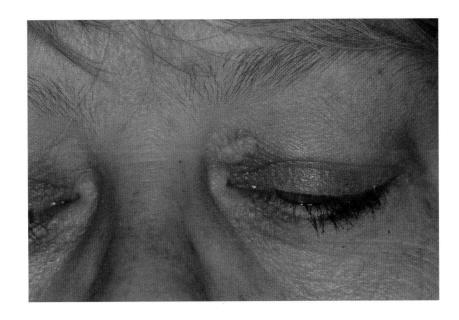

A 47-year-old woman presented with a left upper eyelid lesion. Excisional biopsy of the lesion showed the following histological findings.

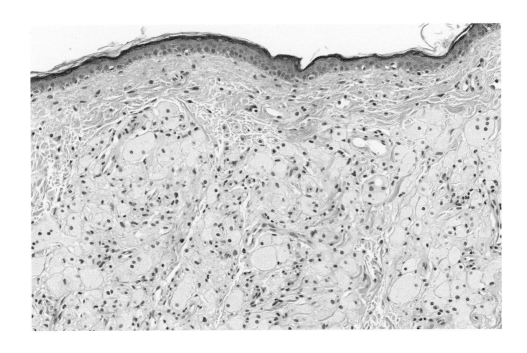

Diagnosis: Xanthelasma.

Clinical description: Clinical examination shows a yellow, elevated lesion on the left upper eyelid.

Histological description: Histopathology reveals a collection of lipid-laden histiocytes within the dermis.

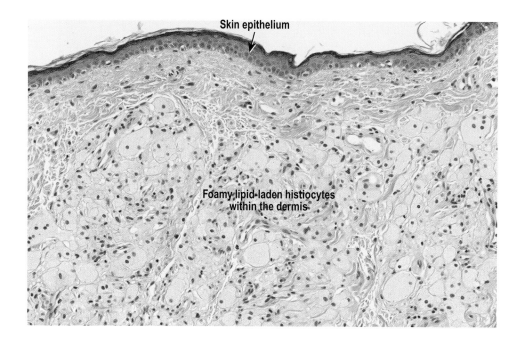

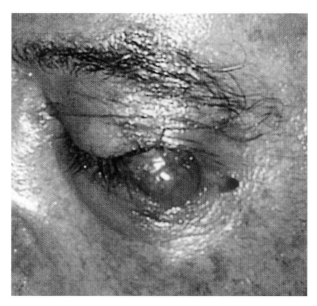

From Albert, Daniel M., Miller, Joan W., Azar, Dimitri T., and Blodi, Barbara A. (eds). 2008. Albert & Jakobiec's Principles and Practice of Ophthalmology, 3rd ed. Philadelphia: Copyright Elsevier 2008.

A 62-year-old man presented with a left lower eyelid lesion.

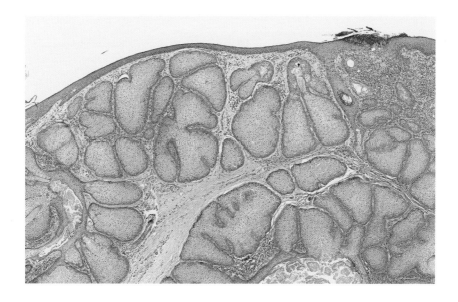

Diagnosis: Sebaceous cell adenoma.

Clinical description: Clinical examination demonstrates a large cystic left lower eyelid lesion.

Histological description: Histopathology demonstrates skin with keratinized squamous epithelium. In the dermis, there are hyperplastic sebaceous glands forming multiple cavities containing proteinaceous material (asterisks). Sebaceous adenoma of the skin may be associated with Muir–Torre syndrome.

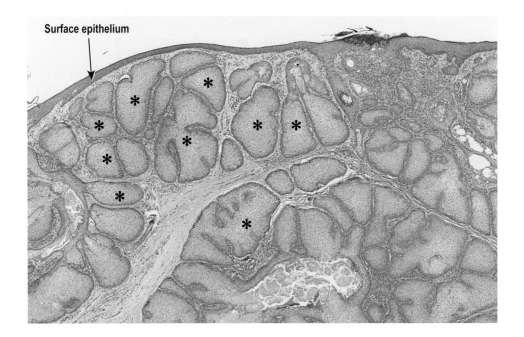

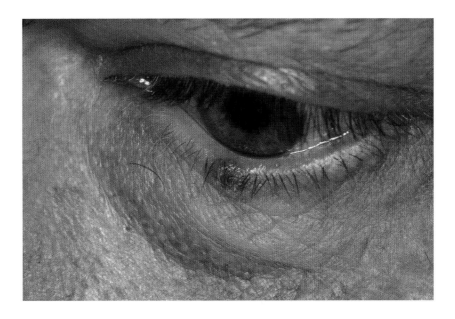

The patient is a 48-year-old man with a 3-month history of a left lower eyelid lesion. The clinical appearance is depicted above.

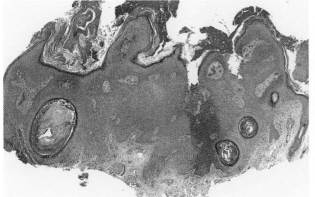
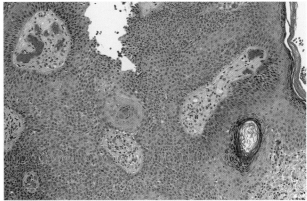

Diagnosis: Inverted follicular keratosis.

Clinical description: External examination reveals a keratinized left lower eyelid mass.

Histological description: The excised lesion demonstrates hyperkeratosis, parakeratosis, and acanthosis. The tissue has an overall inverted papillary pattern. Squamous eddies are seen.

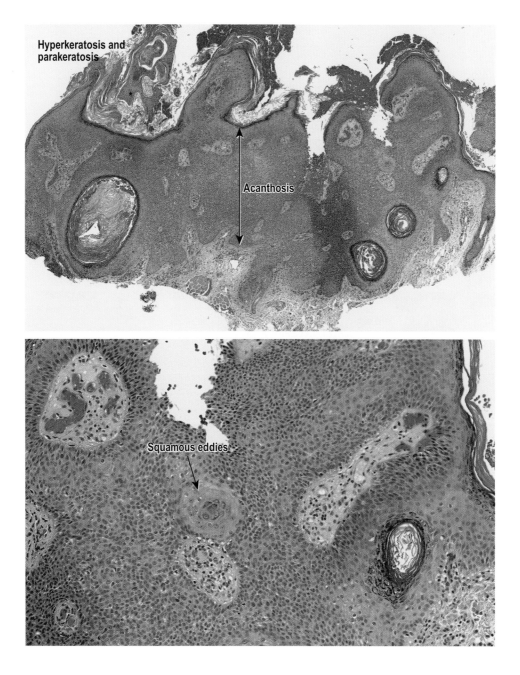

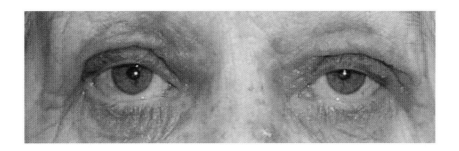

A 74-year-old woman presented with the skin changes seen above.

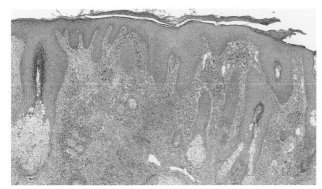 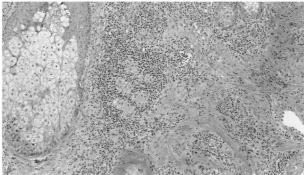

Diagnosis: Rosacea.

Clinical description: Facial and periocular erythema is noted.

Histological description: Histopathology reveals keratinized, stratified squamous epithelium with acanthosis and focal parakeratosis. Granulomatous inflammation surrounding some of the hair follicles is present within the dermis.

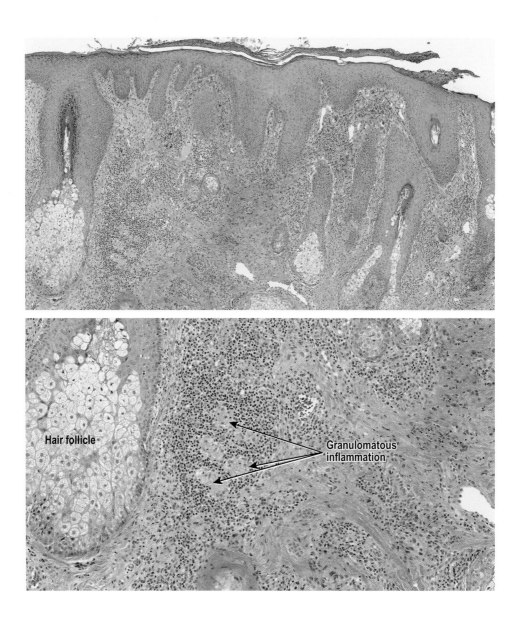

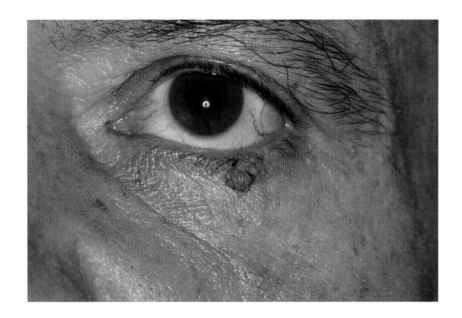

A 57-year-old man presented with multiple pigmented lesions.

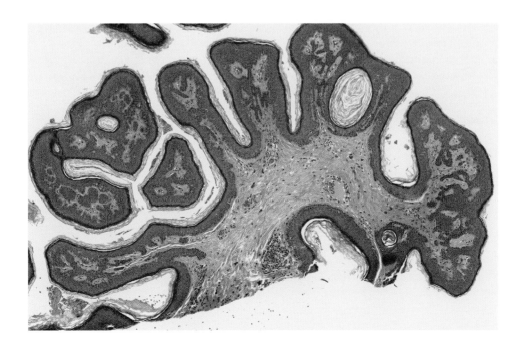

Diagnosis: Seborrheic keratosis (papillomatous).

Clinical description: Multiple brown skin tags in the left lower lid can be seen.

Histological description: Histopathology reveals tissue lined by keratinized stratified squamous epithelium with a few pilosebaceous units and focal basal epithelial pigmentation. There is hyperkeratosis and papillomatous acanthosis. Scattered pseudohorn cysts (asterisks) are also present. Focal areas of chronic inflammation are noted in the dermis.

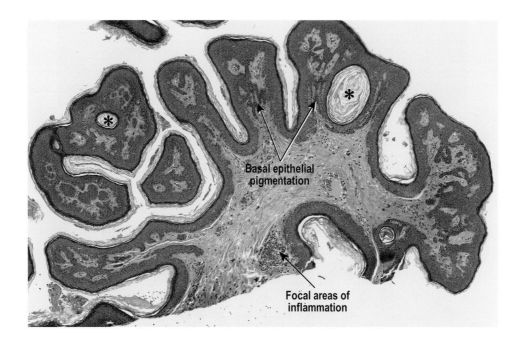

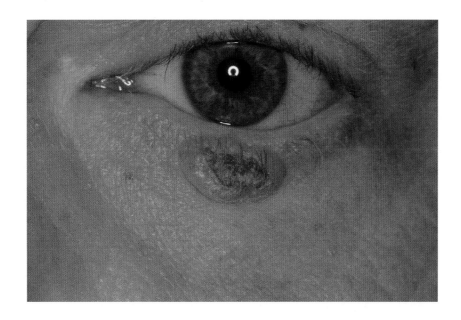

A 53-year-old man presented with a 3-month history of a left lower eyelid lesion.

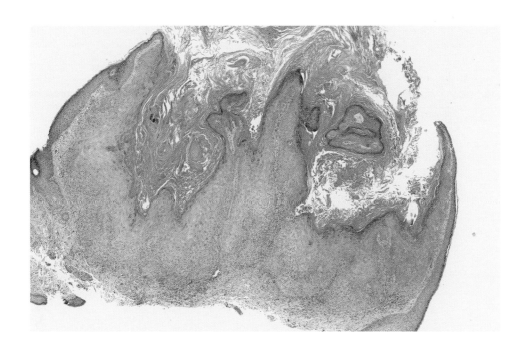

Diagnosis: Keratoacanthoma.

Clinical description: Histopathology reveals a skin lesion with central crater filled with keratin. The edges of the lesion are rolled-up and elevated.

Histological description: Histopathological evaluation reveals a keratinized stratified squamous surface epithelium with a crater-shaped endophytic lesion filled with keratin. Acanthosis and parakeratosis are present. Mild atypia and a few mitotic figures are noted.

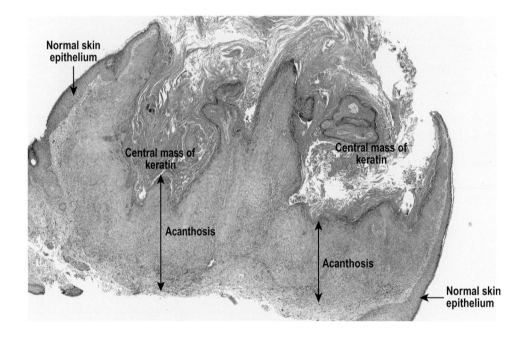

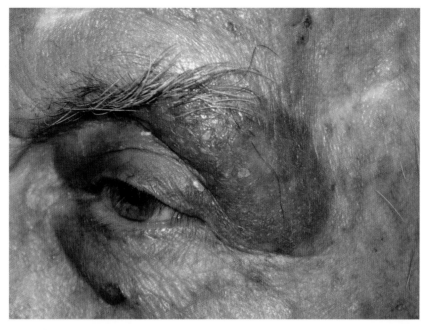

From Albert, Daniel M., Miller, Joan W., Azar, Dimitri T., and Blodi, Barbara A. (eds). 2008. Albert & Jakobiec's Principles and Practice of Ophthalmology, 3rd ed. Philadelphia: Copyright Elsevier 2008.

An 81-year-old man presented with an enlarging lesion on his left brow.

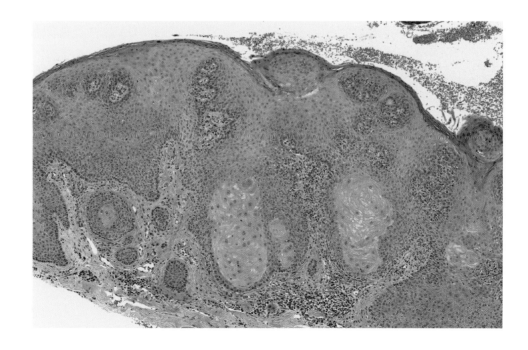

Diagnosis: Squamous cell carcinoma in situ.

Clinical description: Clinical examination reveals an erythematous lesion with scaling.

Histological description: Sections through the specimen show a thickened, keratinized, stratified squamous epithelium with marked hyperkeratosis and parakeratosis. Nests of malignant squamous cells are present (asterisks). Intraepithelial keratin pearls are also seen (short arrow).

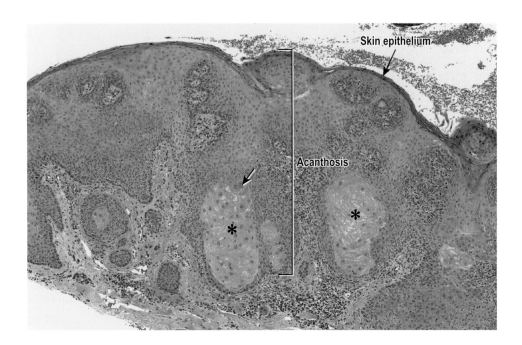

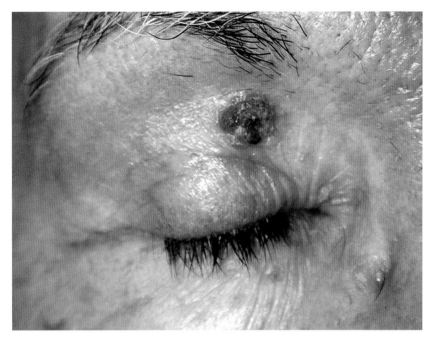

From Albert, Daniel M., Miller, Joan W., Azar, Dimitri T., and Blodi, Barbara A. (eds). 2008. Albert & Jakobiec's Principles and Practice of Ophthalmology, 3rd ed. Philadelphia: Copyright Elsevier. 2008.

A 67-year-old man presented with a 3-month history of an eyelid lesion.

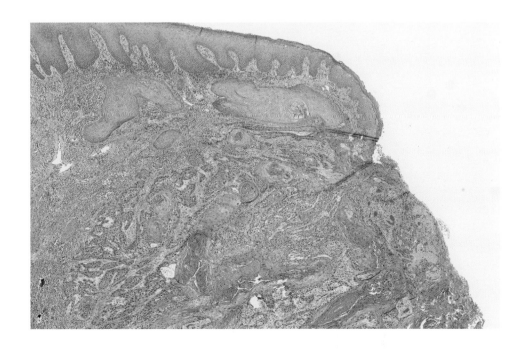

Diagnosis: Invasive squamous cell carcinoma.

Clinical description: Clinical examination reveals an ulcerated and scarred right upper eyelid lesion.

Histological description: Sections through the specimen show keratinized, stratified squamous epithelium. Nests of malignant squamous cells infiltrate the dermis (asterisks). Keratin pearls are also present (arrows).

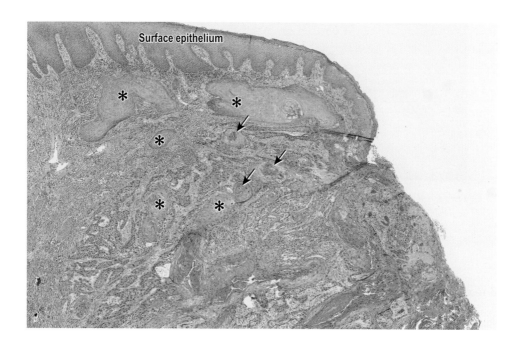

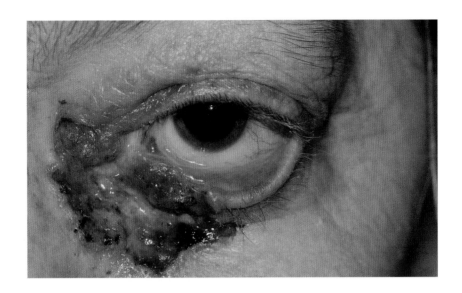

A 69-year-old woman presented with an ulcerated skin lesion. She underwent excisional biopsy.

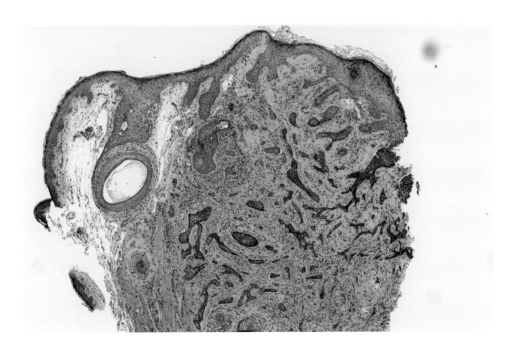

Diagnosis: Morpheaform basal cell carcinoma.

Clinical description: Clinical examination reveals an ulcerated left lower eyelid lesion.

Histological description: Histopathology demonstrates keratinized stratified squamous epithelium overlying a dermis infiltrated with bands and cords of flattened tumor cells.

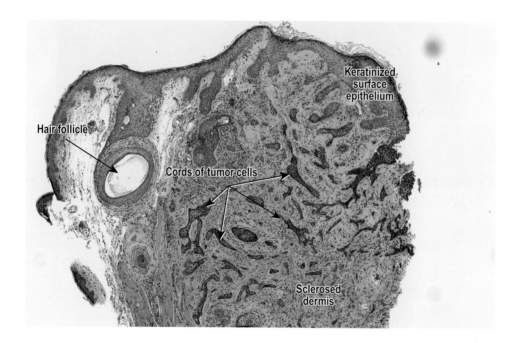

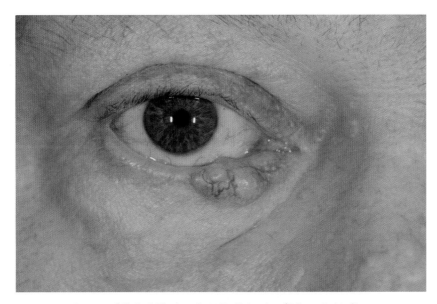

Courtesy of Shahed Ghoghawala M.D. University of Wisconsin-Madison.

A 66-year-old man presented with a right lower eyelid lesion. The lesion had been present for over a year and was increasing in size.

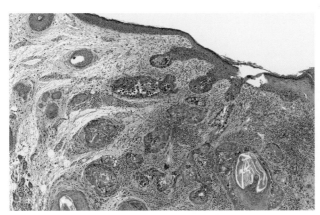

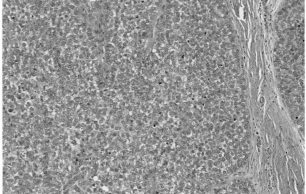

Diagnosis: Sebaceous cell carcinoma with pagetoid spread.

Clinical description: Clinical examination reveals cystic lesions in the right lower eyelid with an associated madarosis.

Histological description: Histopathology reveals tissue lined by keratinized stratified squamous epithelium. Cords and lobules of foamy cells lined by basaloid cells are present within the dermis and subepithelium and infiltrate into the epithelium (pagetoid spread). Higher magnification (bottom) demonstrates the foamy cells in more detail.

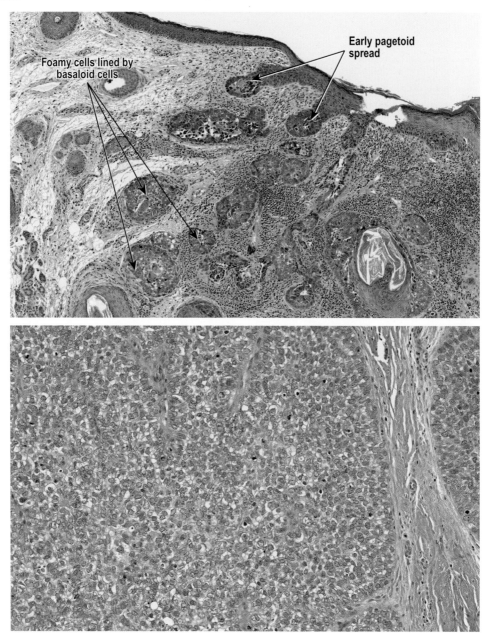

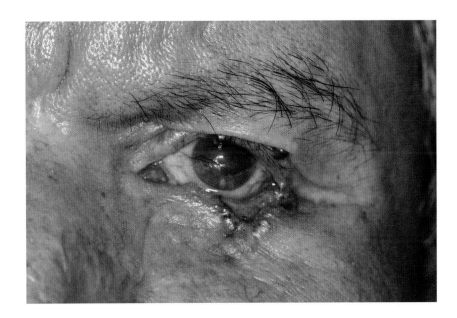

A 65-year-old man presented with several pigmented nodules present on his upper and lower left eyelids.

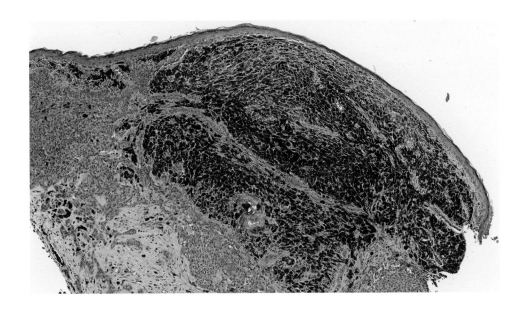

Diagnosis: Pigmented basal cell carcinoma.

Clinical description: Ulcerated left lower eyelid lesion surrounded by a few pigmented nodular lesions is seen. A few pigmented lesions are also present in the left upper eyelid.

Histological description: Histopathology reveals tissue lined by keratinized stratified squamous epithelium. There are extensive islands of atypical basaloid cells with high nuclear to cytoplasmic ratio in the dermis. The islands demonstrate peripheral palisading and retraction artifact (arrow). Dense pigmentation is present. Differentiation from melanoma was confirmed on bleach sections (not shown).

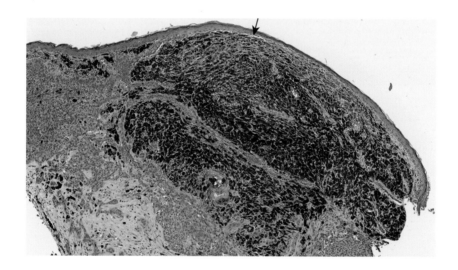

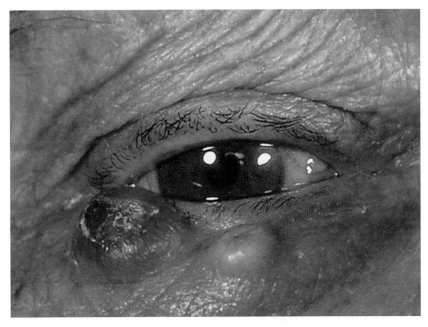

From Albert, Daniel M., Miller, Joan W., Azar, Dimitri T., and Blodi, Barbara A. (eds). 2008. Albert & Jakobiec's Principles and Practice of Ophthalmology, 3rd ed. Philadelphia. Copyright Elsevier 2008.

An 81-year-old man presented with eyelid lesions.

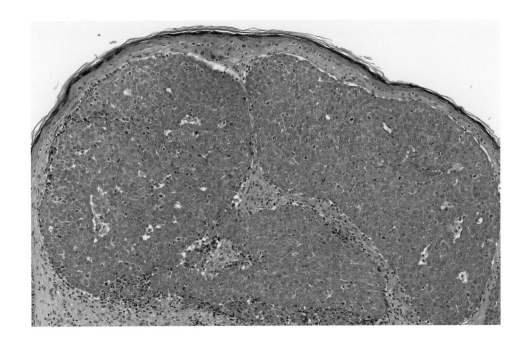

Diagnosis: Merkel cell carcinoma.

Clinical description: Slit-lamp examination demonstrates two elevated eyelid nodules in the right lower lid.

Histological description: Histopathological examination reveals a skin with keratinized stratified squamous epithelium. In the dermis, there are sheets of atypical and pleomorphic cells with finely dispersed chromatin and inconspicuous nucleoli.

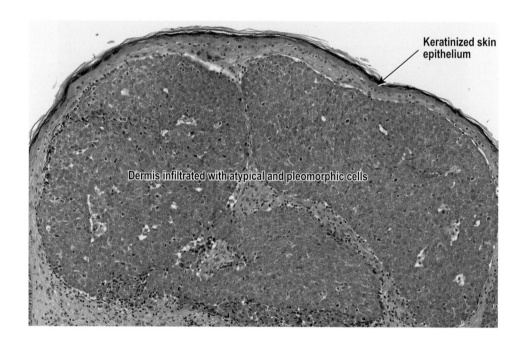

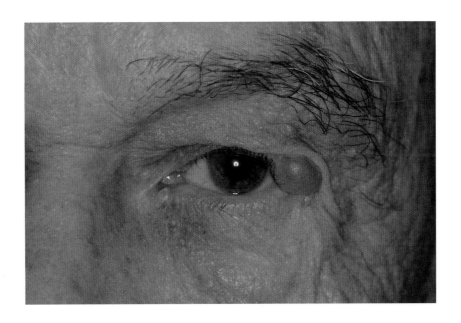

A 72-year-old man presented with a 6-month history of a growing eyelid mass.

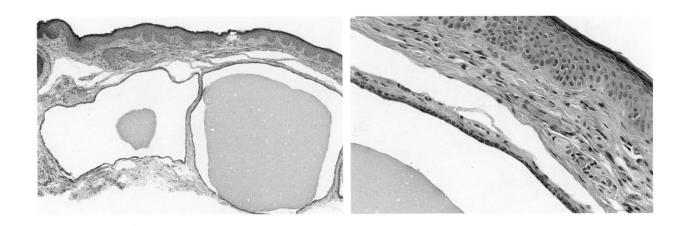

Diagnosis: Eccrine hidrocystoma.

Clinical description: Clinical examination shows a large, translucent fluid-filled eyelid cyst.

Histological description: Multilocular branching lumen (asterisks) filled with eosinophilic material is seen on histopathology. The lumen is lined by a double layer of epithelium. No apical snouts are seen.

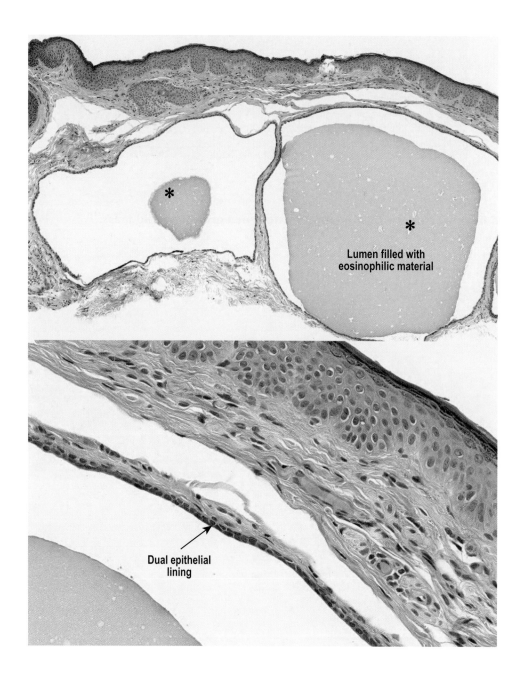

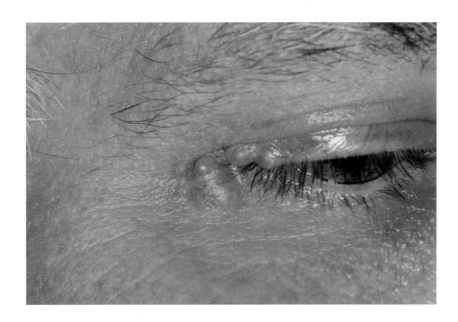

A 53-year-old man presented with multiple cystic lesions in the medial canthus and upper eyelid. He underwent excisional biopsy of the lesions.

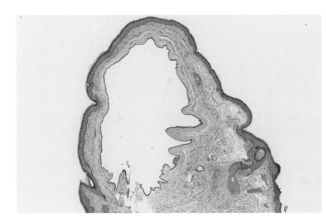

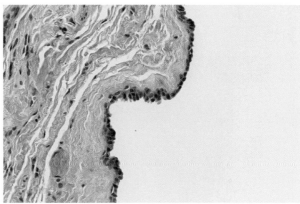

Diagnosis: Apocrine hidrocystoma.

Clinical description: Multiple fluid filled, translucent vesicles in the medial canthus and upper eyelid.

Histological description: Large intradermal cystic cavity lined by a double epithelial layer. The innermost cells display apical snouts (decapitation bodies).

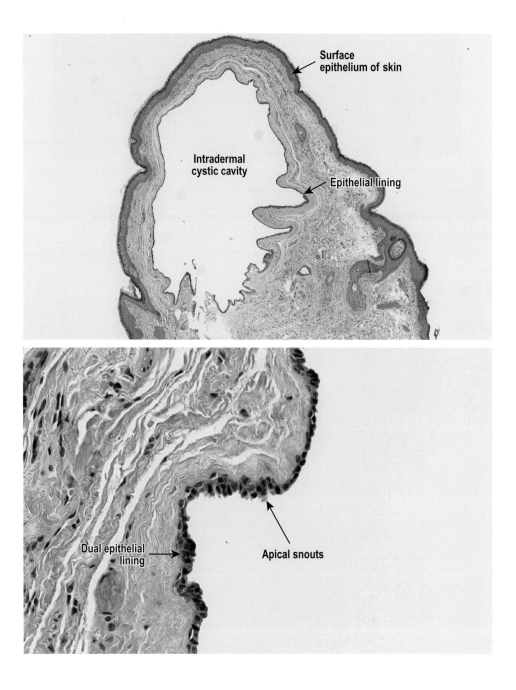

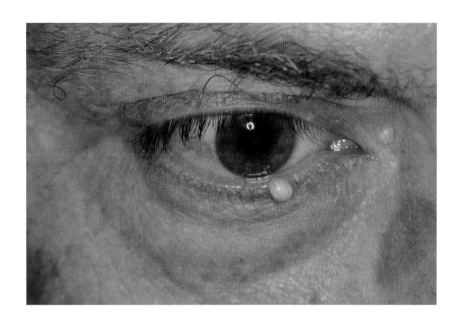

A 58-year-old man presented with a slow-growing right lower eyelid lesion. He later underwent an excisional biopsy of the lesion.

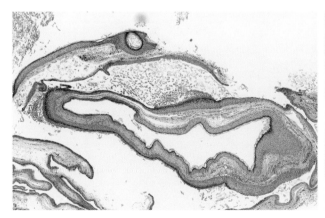
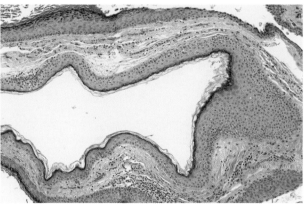

Diagnosis: Epithelial inclusion cyst.

Clinical description: Raised white/opaque lesion is seen in the right lower eyelid margin.

Histological description: Large cystic space lined by keratinized stratified squamous epithelium is seen within the dermis. Unlike dermoid cysts, the epithelial lining does not have pilosebaceous units.

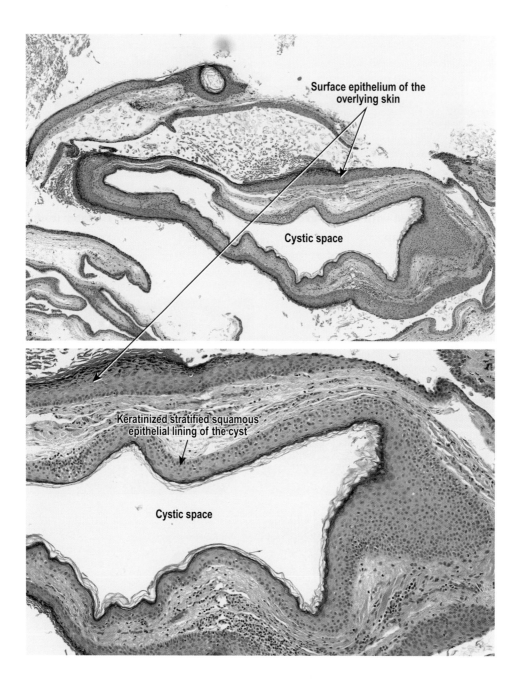

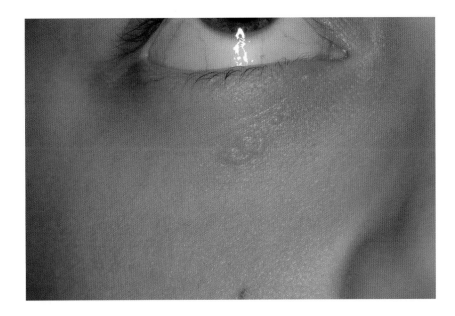

The patient is a 21-year-old woman who presented with multiple skin lesions under the right lower eyelid.

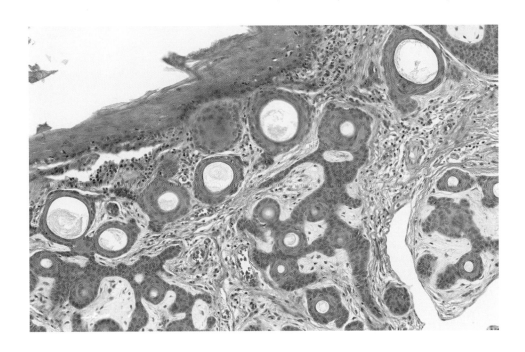

Diagnosis: Syringoma.

Clinical description: Multiple flesh-colored skin lesions are seen.

Histological description: Histopathology reveals keratinized stratified squamous epithelium overlying numerous single and double-layered epithelial strands with cysts (asterisks) and some with "tadpole configuration" (arrowheads) present throughout the dermis.

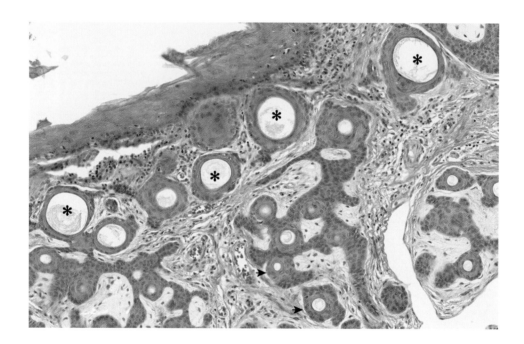

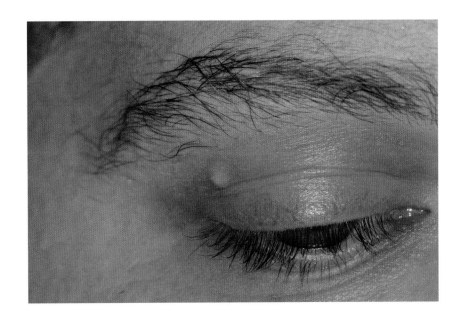

A 35-year-old woman presented with a 3-month history of an eyelid lesion.

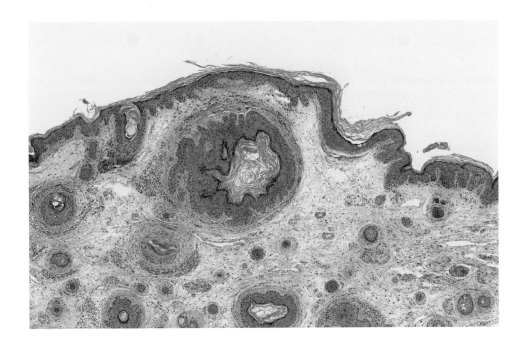

Diagnosis: Infundibular cyst.

Clinical description: Clinical examination reveals a subcutaneous mass in the right upper eyelid.

Histological description: The slides reveal tissue lined by a keratinized stratified squamous epithelium. A follicular infundibular structure, filled with keratin, is seen within the dermis (circle).

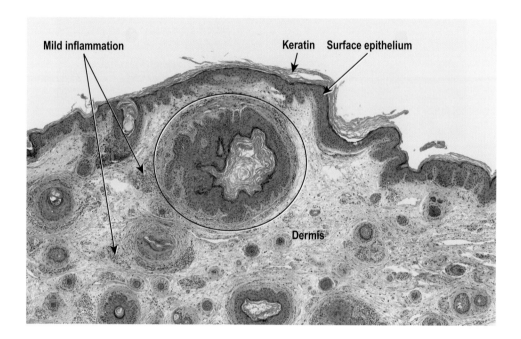

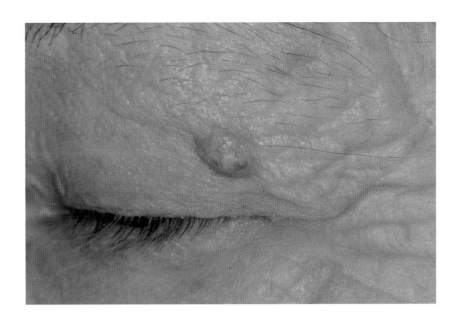

An 84-year-old female presented with a 6-month history of a left upper eyelid lesion.

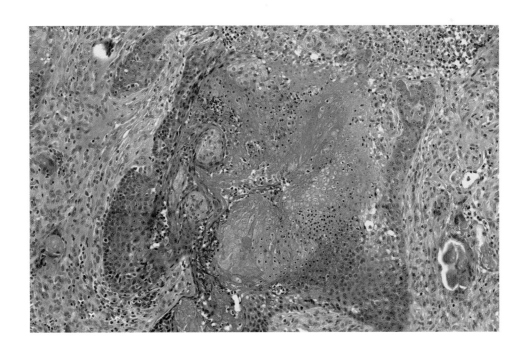

Diagnosis: Pilomatrixoma.

Clinical description: A raised, nodular lesion, with a few dilated vessels, is seen in the left upper eyelid.

Histological description: Histopathology demonstrates islands of shadow cells and basophilic cells intermixed with numerous epithelioid histiocytes. Calcium is present.

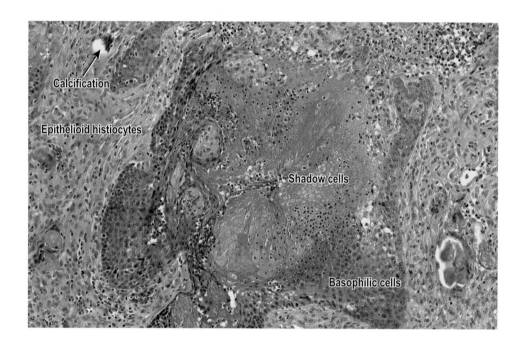

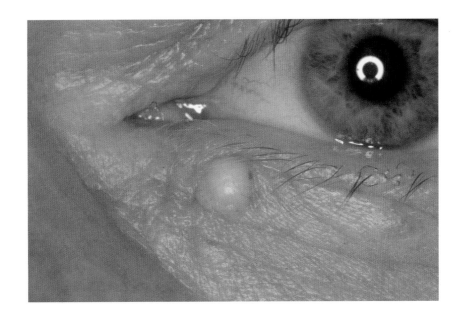

A 76-year-old woman presented with a rapidly growing left lower eyelid lesion.

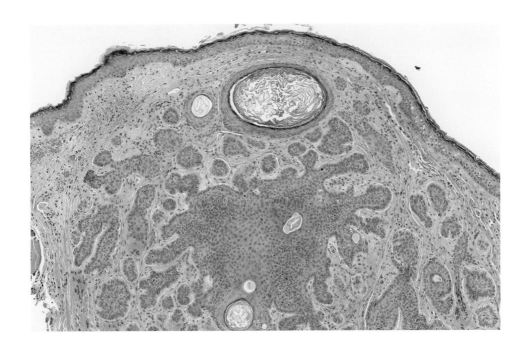

Diagnosis: Trichoepithelioma.

Clinical description: A raised pearly lesion with a smooth surface is noted.

Histological description: The slides reveal stratified squamous epithelium overlying a dermis with multiple small nests of basaloid cells with peripheral palisading of their nuclei (asterisks).

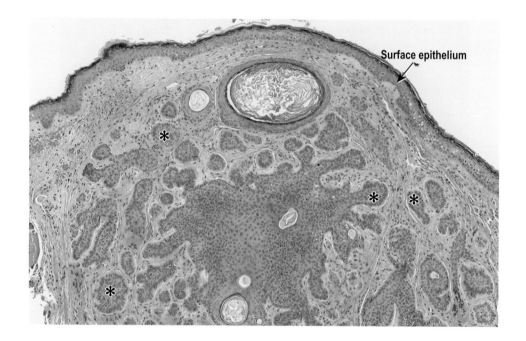

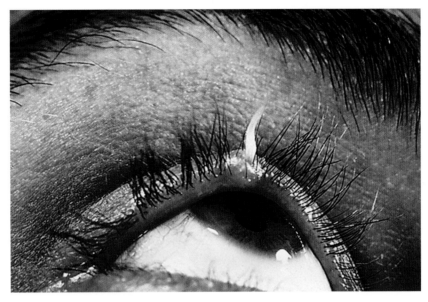

From Albert, Daniel M., Miller, Joan W., Azar, Dimitri T., and Blodi, Barbara A. (eds). 2008. Albert & Jakobiec's Principles and Practice of Ophthalmology, 3rd ed. Philadelphia: Copyright Elsevier 2008.

A 35-year-old woman presented with a 3-month history of an eyelid lesion.

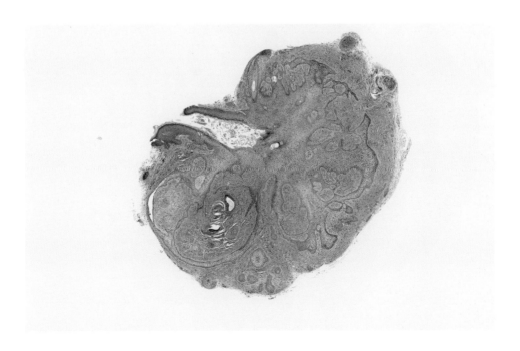

Diagnosis: Trichofolliculoma.

Clinical description: Clinical examination reveals a cystic lesion in the right upper eyelid with a wisp of lanugo hairs emanating from it.

Histological description: The slides reveal tissue lined by a keratinized stratified squamous epithelium. A follicular infundibular structure, surrounded by multiple small follicles (asterisks), containing keratin, and communicating with the skin surface can be seen.

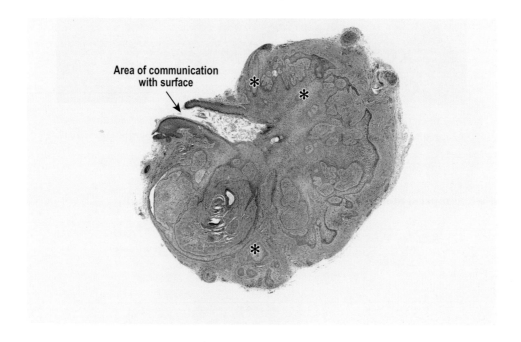

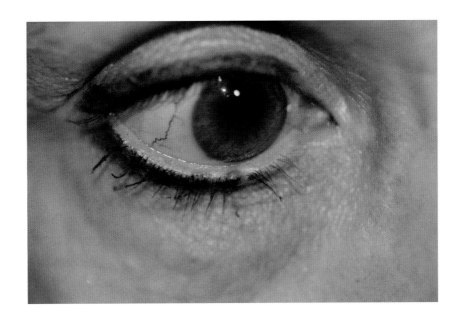

A 43-year-old woman presented with a nodular right lower eyelid lesion.

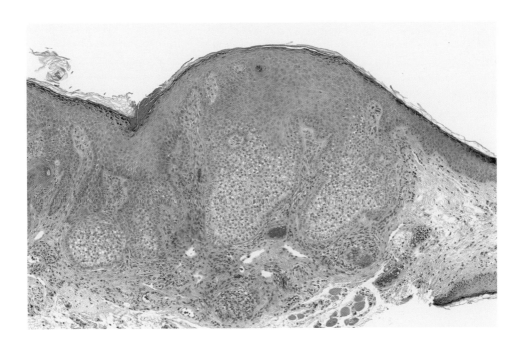

Diagnosis: Trichilemmoma.

Clinical description: Clinical examination reveals a round, nodular, flesh-colored right lower eyelid skin lesion.

Histological description: The histopathology reveals hyperkeratotic stratified squamous epithelium with marked parakeratosis and acanthosis. Areas of well-defined and plate-like clear cells (asterisk) and epithelial down-growth into the dermis are seen. Areas of palisading are also seen.

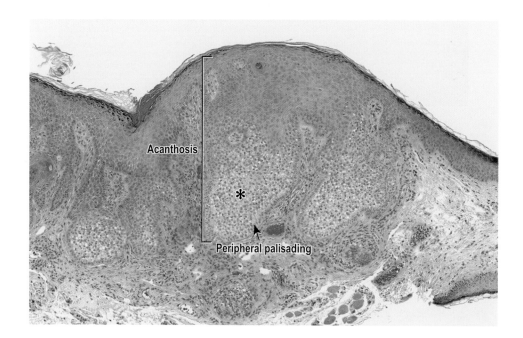

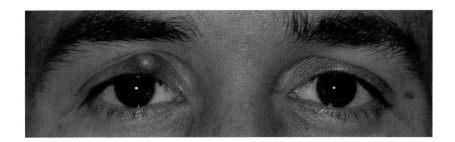

An 18-year-old man presented with a 1-week history of a right upper eyelid nodule refractory to treatment with warm compress and eyelid massage.

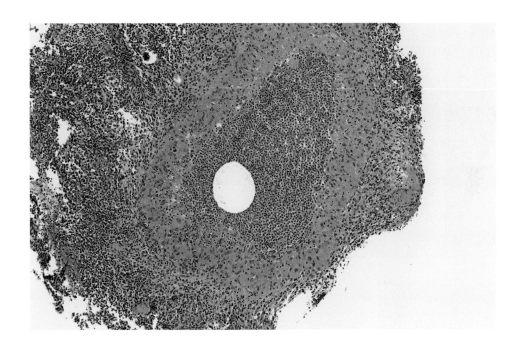

Diagnosis: Chalazion.

Clinical description: A red, elevated right upper eyelid mass is seen.

Histological description: Granulomatous and nongranulomatous chronic inflammation is seen surrounding a large lipid vacuole. Multinucleated giant cells are also seen.

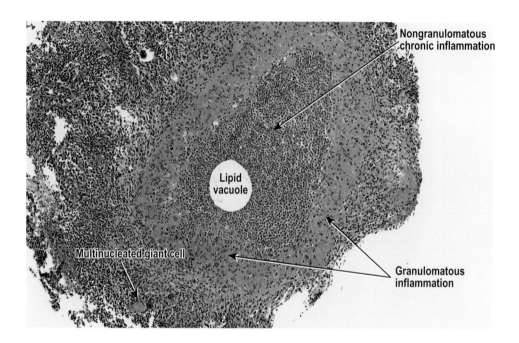

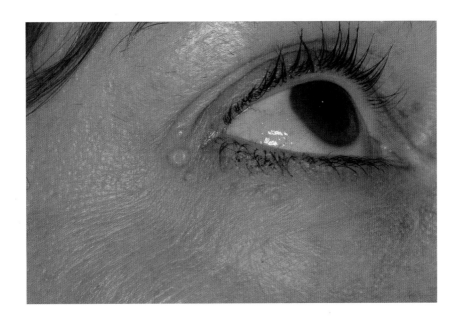

A 38-year-old woman presented with multiple eyelid skin lesions.

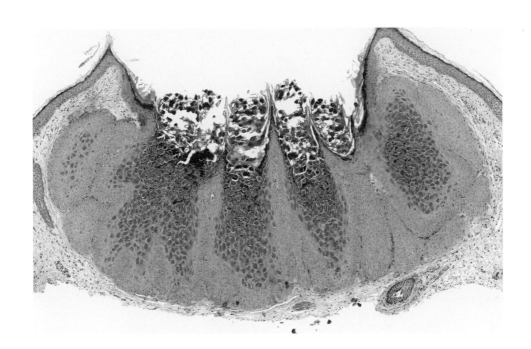

Diagnosis: Molluscum contagiosum.

Clinical description: Clinical examination reveals multiple pearly flesh-colored dome-shaped lesions.

Histological description: Histopathology reveals a discrete dome-shaped lesion with an umbilicated center. Pear-shaped acanthotic lobules of epithelial cells filled with eosinophilic intracytoplasmic inclusion bodies (Henderson–Patterson corpuscles) are seen. The inclusion bodies (circles) are deeply eosinophilic in the lower cells and become less eosinophilic towards the level of the granular layer.

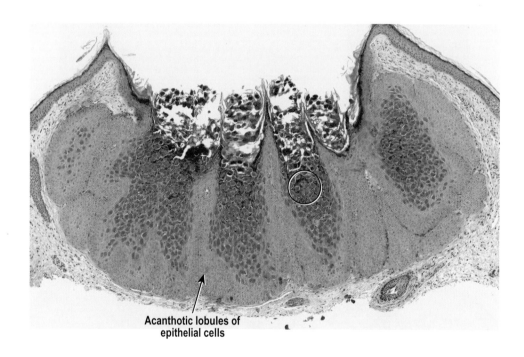

Acanthotic lobules of
epithelial cells

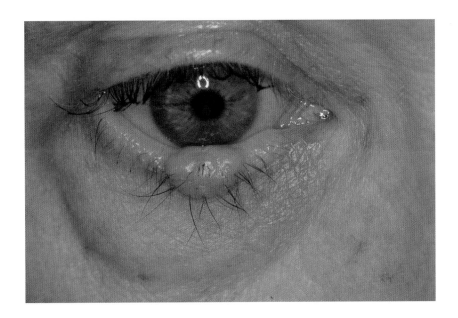

A 58-year-old woman presented with a right lower eyelid lesion. Excisional biopsy of the lesion shows the following histological findings.

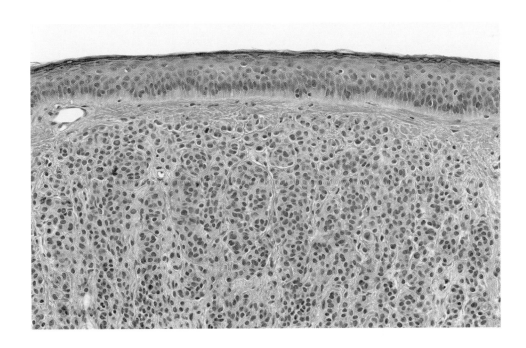

Diagnosis: Intradermal nevus.

Clinical description: Clinical examination reveals a pearly, flesh-colored, well-circumscribed raised lesion.

Histological description: Histopathology reveals nests of benign melanocytic cells confined to the dermis. A cell free region known as the "grenz zone" is seen beneath the epithelium.

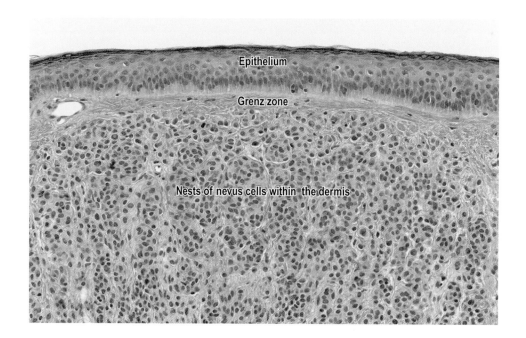

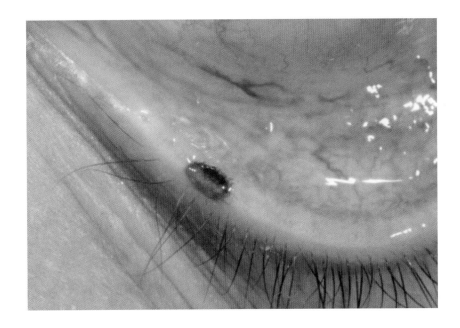

A 33-year-old woman presented with an eyelid lesion. The lesion was removed and evaluated histopathologically.

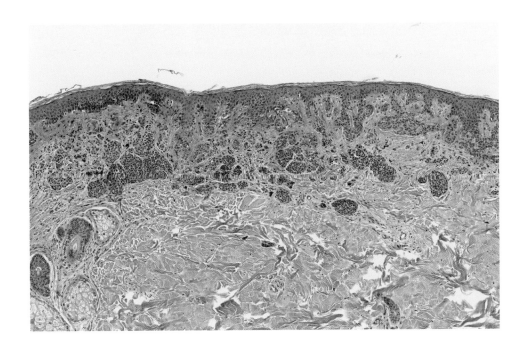

Diagnosis: Compound nevus.

Clinical description: A mostly flat, darkly pigmented lesion at the margin of the left lower eyelid is noted.

Histological description: Nests and nodules of ovoid basaloid cells are present within the dermis as well as at the junction between the epidermis and the dermis.

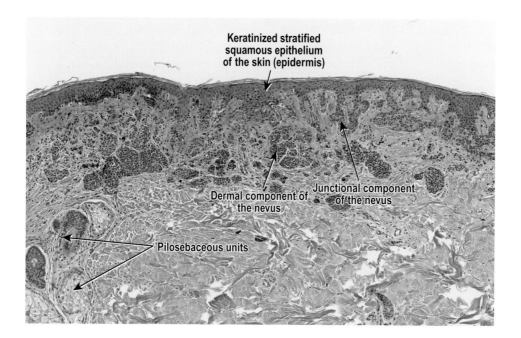

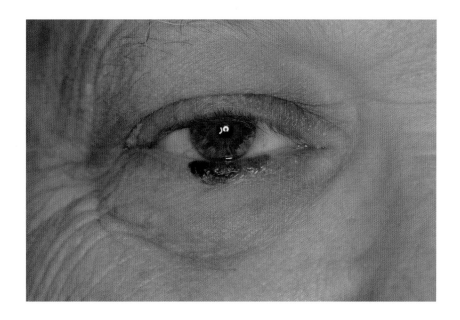

A 62-year-old woman presented with a pigmented lesion in the right lower eyelid.

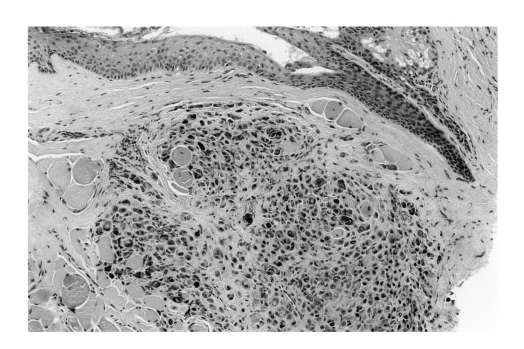

Diagnosis: Malignant melanoma of the eyelid.

Clinical description: Clinical examination reveals a slightly raised pigmented skin lesion.

Histological description: Histopathology demonstrates skin infiltrated with pigmented atypical melanocytes (arrows) consistent with melanoma.

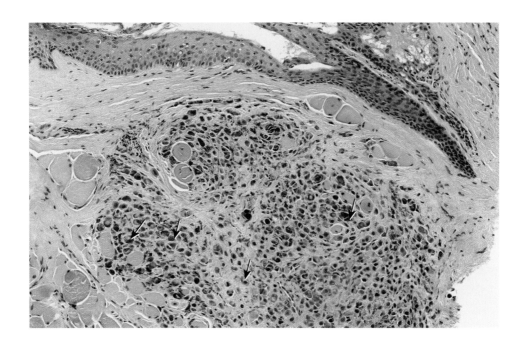

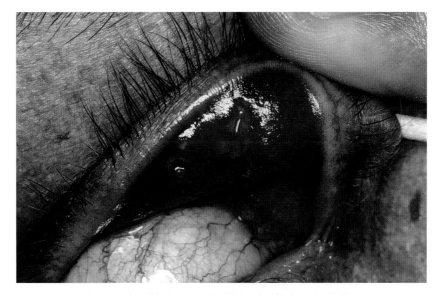

Courtesy of Neal P. Barney, M.D. University of Wisconsin-Madison

A 44-year-old obese male presented with dry, irritated eyes.

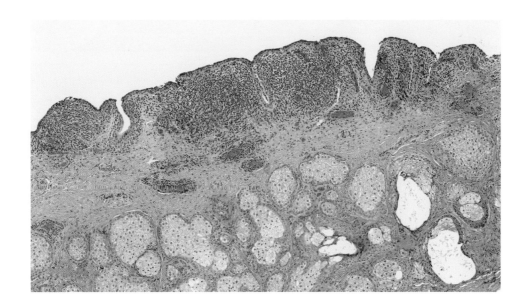

Diagnosis: Floppy eyelid syndrome.

Clinical description: Upper eyelid laxity is apparent. The tarsal conjunctiva has a velvety appearance.

Histological description: Biopsy shows multiple conjunctival papillae marked by elevated nodules infiltrated with inflammatory cells (arrows) and containing fronds of vascular core (arrowheads).

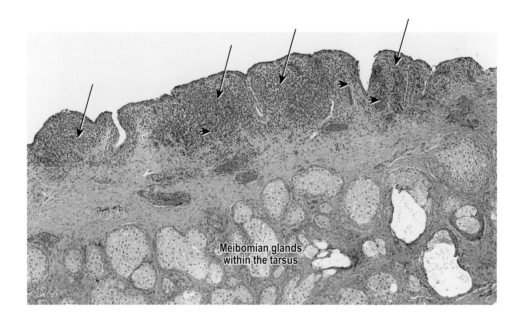

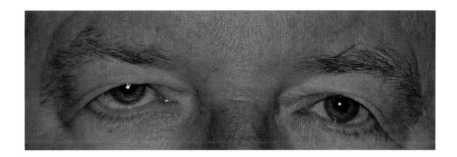

A 63-year-old man presented with a chief complaint of droopy eyelids. He underwent a functional blepharoplasty.

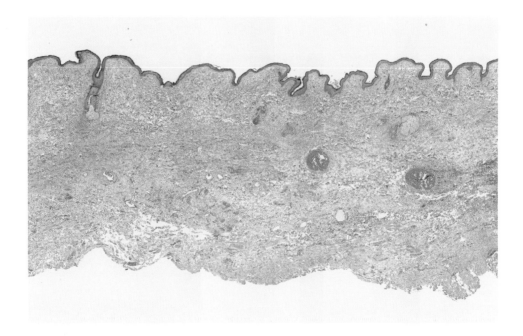

Diagnosis: Dermatochalasis.

Clinical description: Bilateral ptosis and redundancy of the upper eyelid skin is noted on clinical examination.

Histological description: Histopathology reveals keratinized stratified squamous epithelium with associated pilosebaceous units overlying a dermis with loosely arranged collagen fibers.

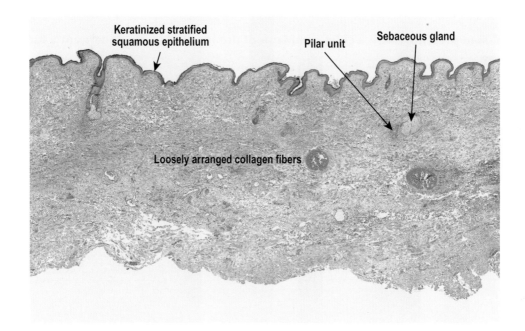

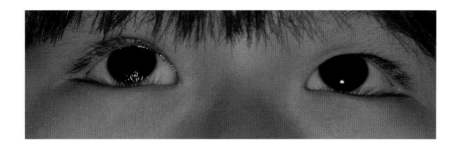

A 3-year-old child was brought in by his mother for evaluation of abnormal eyelids.

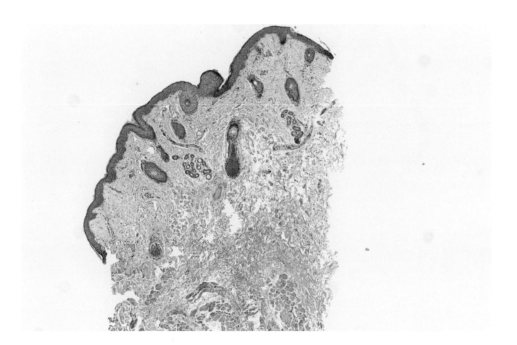

Diagnosis: Entropion with normal histology.

Clinical description: Clinical examination demonstrates bilateral lower eyelid entropion.

Histological description: The slides reveal tissue lined by keratinized stratified squamous epithelium with associated pilosebaceous units, muscle, and fat (normal skin).

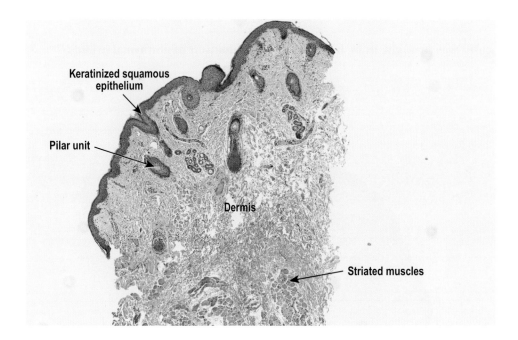

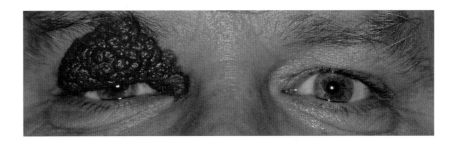

A 44-year-old man presented with an eyelid lesion. The lesion had been present for many years causing severe ptosis.

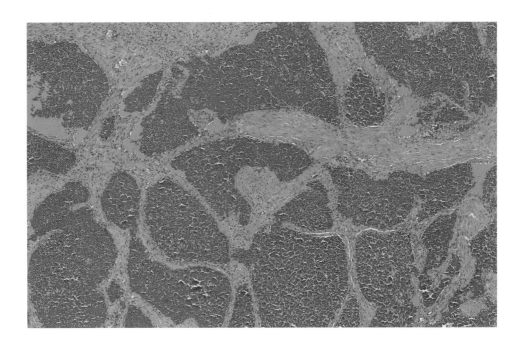

Diagnosis: Cavernous hemangioma of the eyelid.

Clinical description: Clinical examination shows a corrugated, reddish-purple elevated right upper eyelid lesion.

Histological description: Histopathology shows large, dilated vascular channels that are lined by a single layer of flat endothelium. The vascular channels are filled with red blood cells.

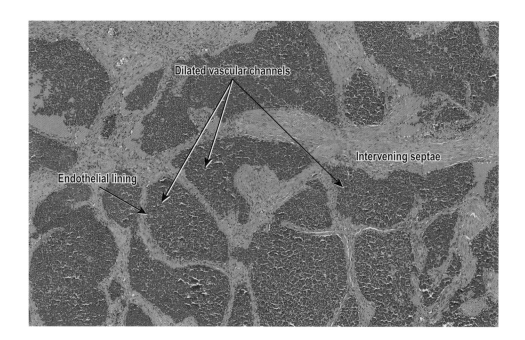

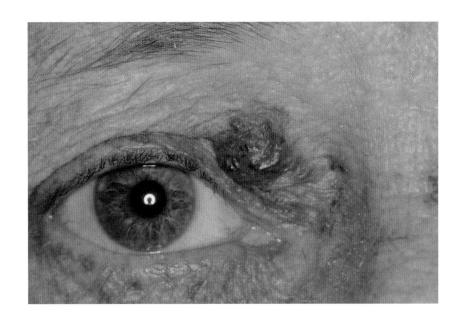

The patient is a 58-year-old woman who presented with a right upper eyelid lesion.

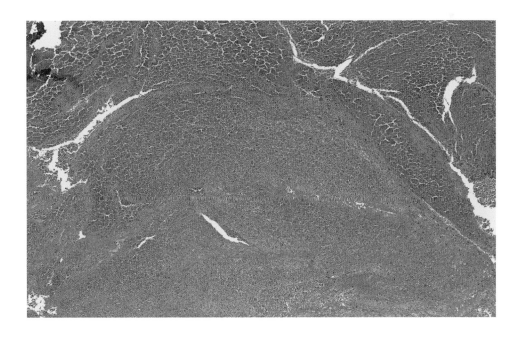

Diagnosis: Eyelid varix.

Clinical description: Clinical examination reveals a vascular cutaneous lesion on the right upper eyelid.

Histological description: Histopathology demonstrates a few thin-walled dilated vascular channels lined by a monolayer of endothelial cells and filled with red blood cells.

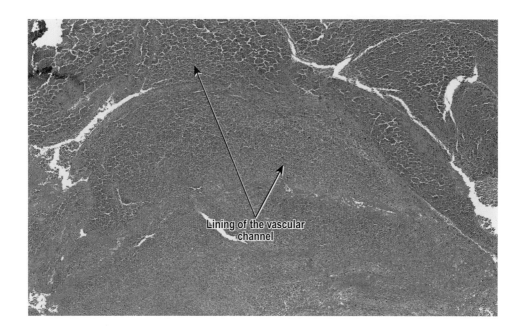

Lining of the vascular channel

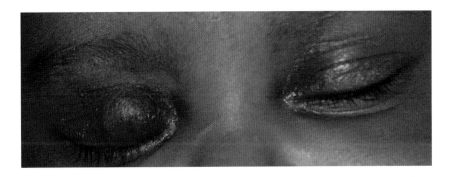

A 2-year-old infant has had the eyelid finding shown above since birth. He later underwent an excisional biopsy of the right upper eyelid lesion.

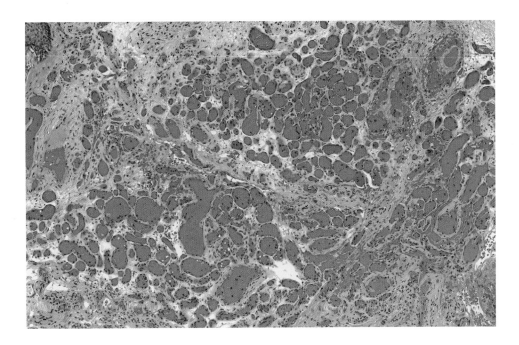

Diagnosis: Eyelid capillary hemangioma.

Clinical description: An elevated reddish right upper eyelid swelling is seen.

Histological description: Proliferation of lobulated capillaries, lined by a single layer of endothelial cells is seen within the dermis. The capillaries are separated by fibrous septae.

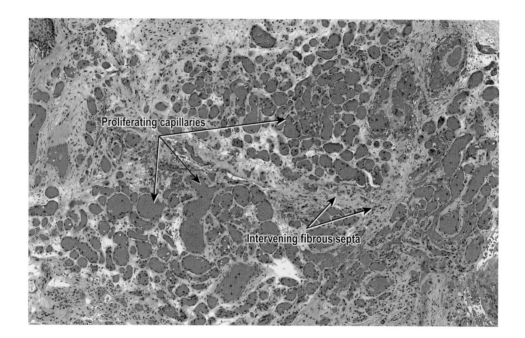

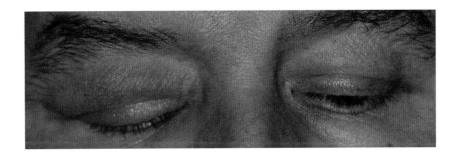

A 48-year-old man presented with redness and swelling of his right upper eyelid. He underwent excisional biopsy of the eyelid.

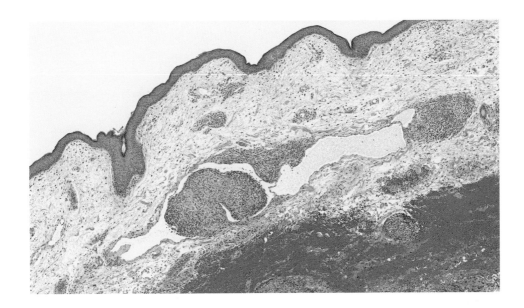

Diagnosis: Melkersson–Rosenthal syndrome.

Clinical description: Right upper eyelid edema and erythema is noted.

Histological description: Histopathology demonstrates skin tissue lined by keratinized stratified squamous epithelium. Granulomatous inflammation is seen within the blood vessel lumen, a finding that is consistent with Melkersson–Rosenthal syndrome.

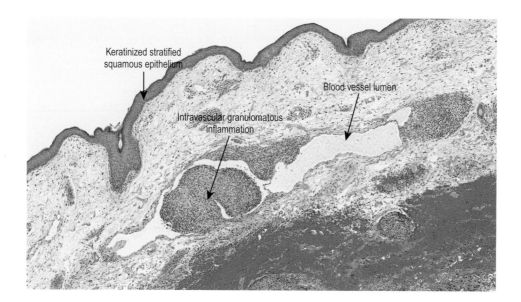

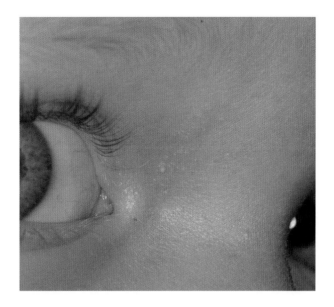

A 2-year-old child presented with yellowish skin lesions present since birth.

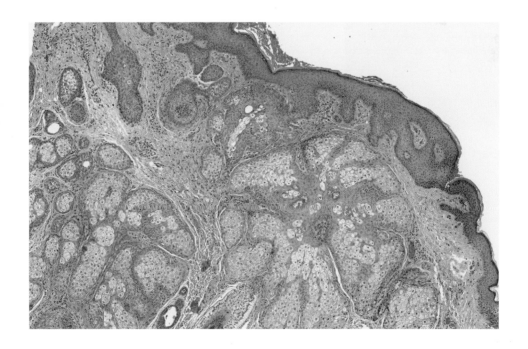

Diagnosis: Nevus sebaceous.

Clinical description: Clinical examination reveals multiple elevated and flat skin lesions above the medial canthus.

Histological description: Histopathology reveals tissue lined by a keratinized stratified squamous epithelium with associated hair follicles and numerous sebaceous glands. The lesion is hyperkeratotic, acanthotic, and papillomatous with focal areas of parakeratosis.

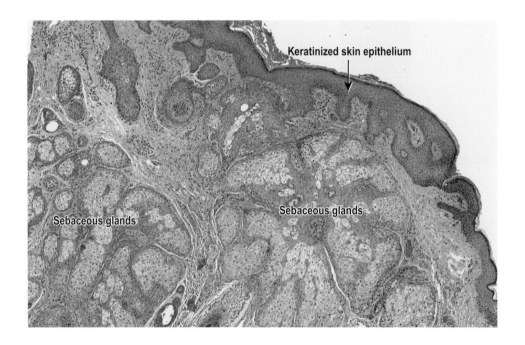

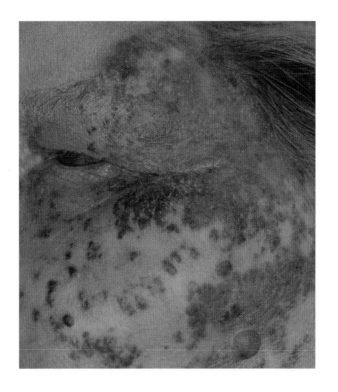

A 64-year-old woman presented with multiple lesions on her face.

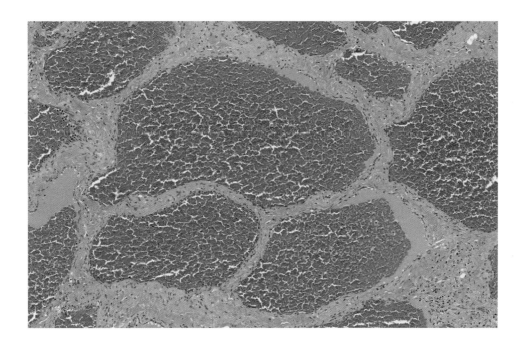

Diagnosis: Face and eyelid cavernous hemangioma.

Clinical description: Clinical examination reveals multiple flat and elevated vascular and pigmented skin lesions.

Histological description: Histopathological evaluation reveals lobules of blood-filled dilated vascular channels lined by a flat endothelial layer.

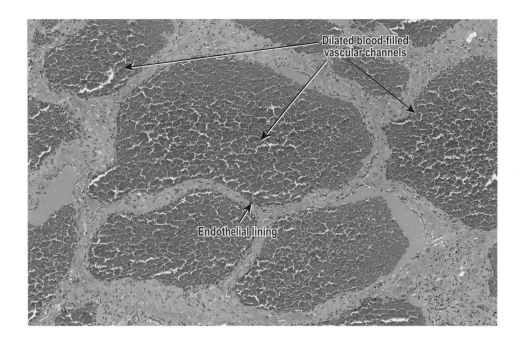

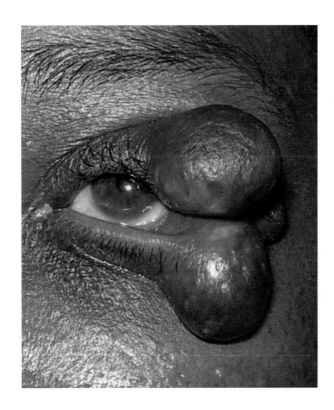

A 56-year-old man presented with a growing eyelid mass. He later underwent excisional biopsy of the eyelid lesions.

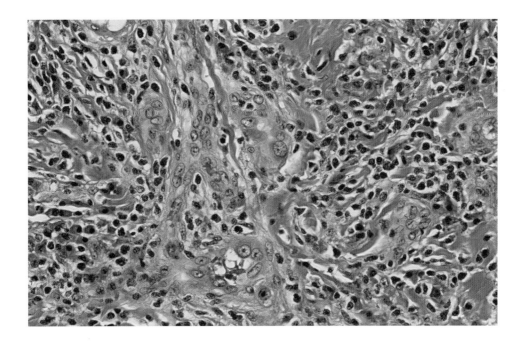

Diagnosis: Angiolymphoid hyperplasia with eosinophilia (ALHE).

Clinical description: Clinical examination reveals round, flesh-colored growths over the upper and lower eyelids.

Histological description: Histopathology reveals vascular proliferation (asterisks) with vessels demonstrating intracytoplasmic vacuolization of their endothelium (arrowheads). Numerous eosinophils, plasma cells, and lymphocytes are also seen.

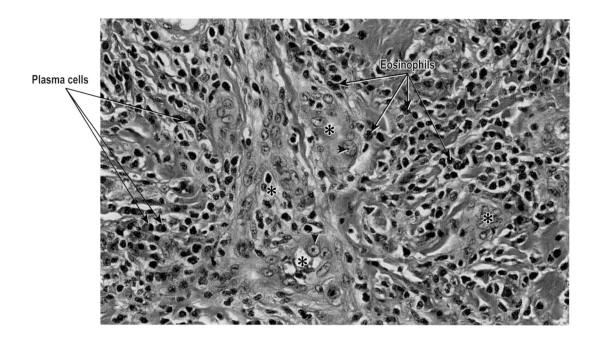

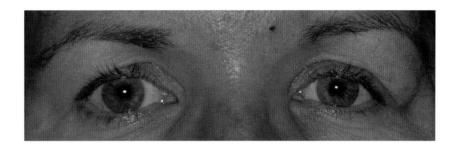

A 45-year-old woman presented with left upper eyelid fullness. Excisional biopsy of the lesion shows the histological findings shown below.

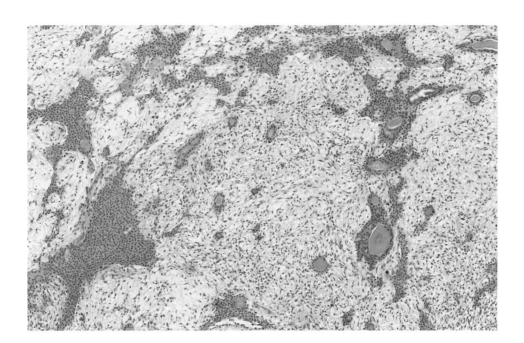

Diagnosis: Pleomorphic adenoma (benign mixed tumor).

Clinical description: Mild fullness of the left upper eyelid is noted.

Histological description: The tumor contains ductules and mesenchymal elements. The ductules are composed of dual epithelial layers. There is differentiation of the outer epithelial layer into mesenchymal elements such as fat, cartilage, and bone.

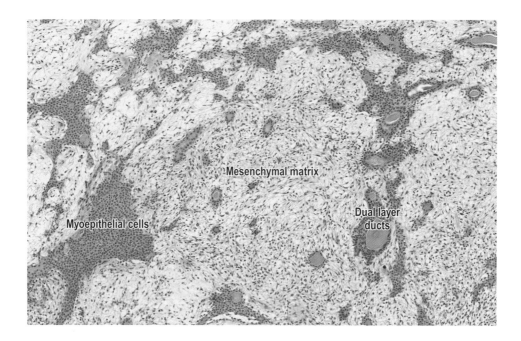

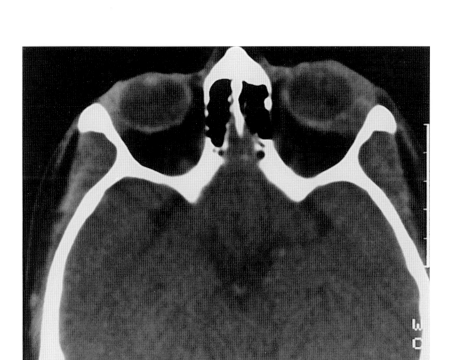

From Albert, Daniel M., Miller, Joan W., Azar, Dimitri T., and Blodi, Barbara A. (eds). 2008. Albert & Jakobiec's Principles and Practice of Ophthalmology, 3rd ed. Philadelphia: Copyright Elsevier 2008.

A 34-year-old woman presented with pain and swelling of her left upper eyelid for the past week. The patient's CT scan is shown above.

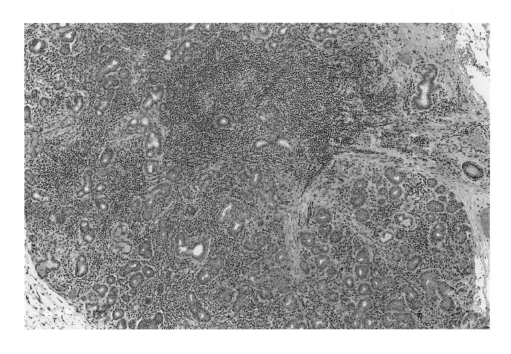

Diagnosis: Dacryoadenitis.

Clinical description: A CT scan of the orbit shows enlargement of the lacrimal gland consistent with dacryoadenitis.

Histological description: Histopathology reveals lacrimal gland tissue that contains aggregates of chronic nongranulomatous, lymphocytic inflammation without necrosis (circles). CD3 and CD20 staining do not show monoclonality (not shown).

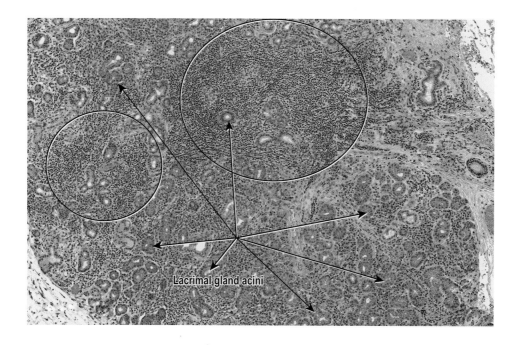

Lacrimal gland acini

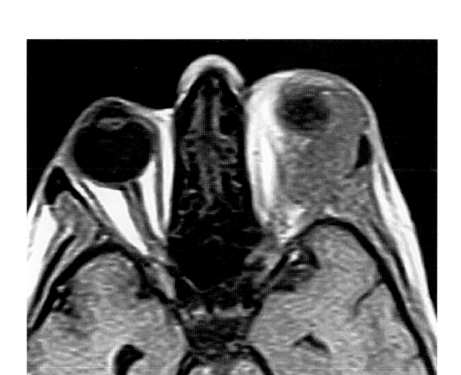

From Albert, Daniel M., Miller, Joan W., Azar, Dimitri T., and Blodi, Barbara A. (eds). 2008. Albert & Jakobiec's Principles and Practice of Ophthalmology, 3rd ed. Philadelphia: Copyright Elsevier 2008.

A 68-year-old patient presented with pain, diplopia, and proptosis. The patient's MRI is shown above.

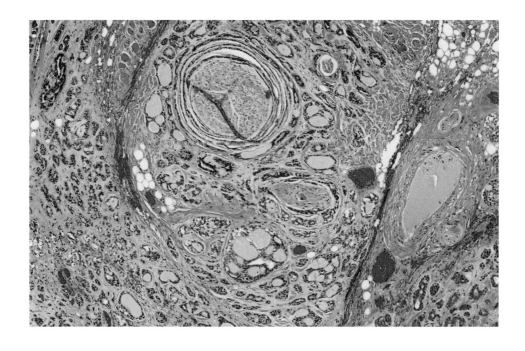

Diagnosis: Adenoid cystic carcinoma.

Clinical description: Magnetic resonance imaging shows a left orbital tumor with erosion of the left lateral orbital wall.

Histological description: Histopathology demonstrates tumor with classic "Swiss cheese" pattern, consisting of cysts (asterisks) surrounded by basaloid cells (arrows). The tumor demonstrates perineural invasion.

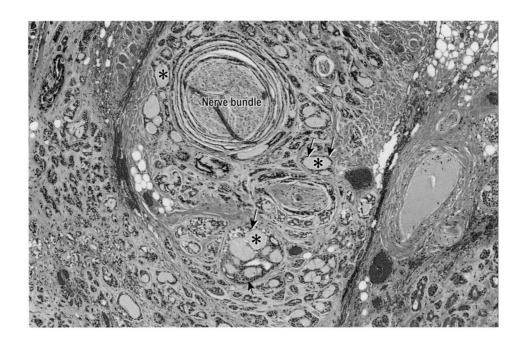

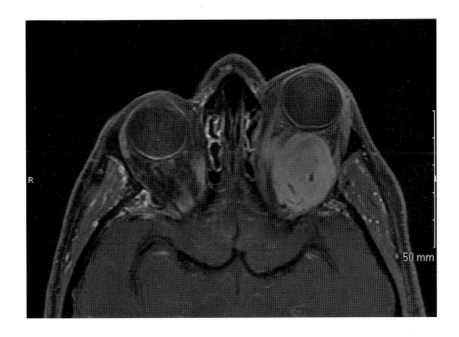

A 59-year-old man presented with double vision and left eye proptosis.

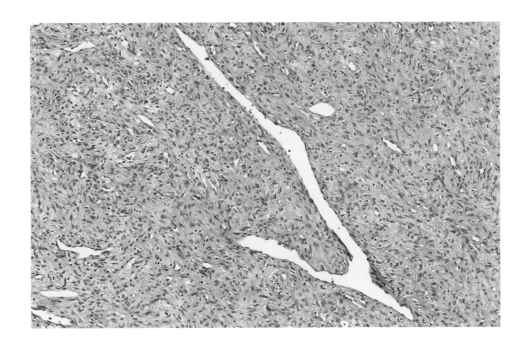

Diagnosis: Hemangiopericytoma.

Clinical description: A well-circumscribed intraconal mass is seen on MRI.

Histological description: The histopathology reveals dilated vascular channels with a "staghorn" configuration within a cellular matrix composed of proliferated pericytes.

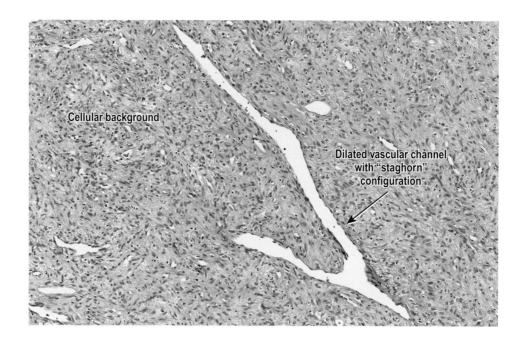

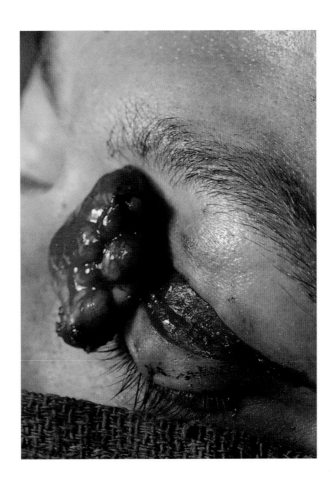

A 21-year-old man presented with increasing proptosis over the past 6 months. The photograph above was taken during an orbital biopsy.

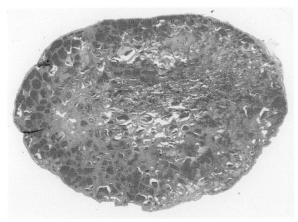

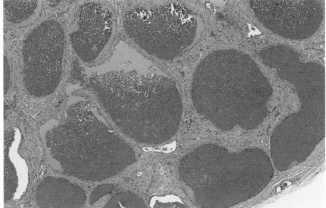

Diagnosis: Cavernous hemangioma of the orbit.

Clinical description: The intraoperative photograph demonstrates a well-circumscribed, vascular orbital lesion.

Histological description: Histopathology demonstrates well-circumscribed lesions composed of dilated thick-walled blood vessels lined by endothelium. The vascular spaces are filled with blood.

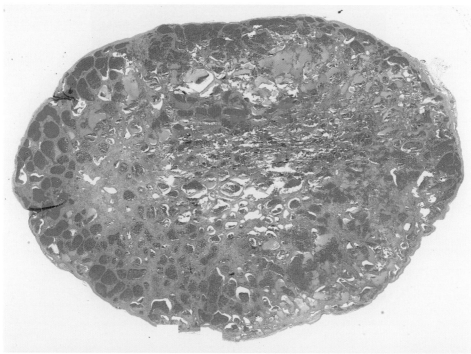

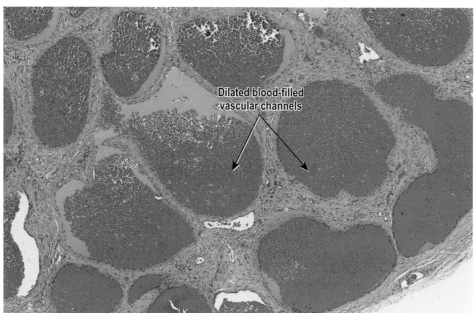

Dilated blood-filled vascular channels

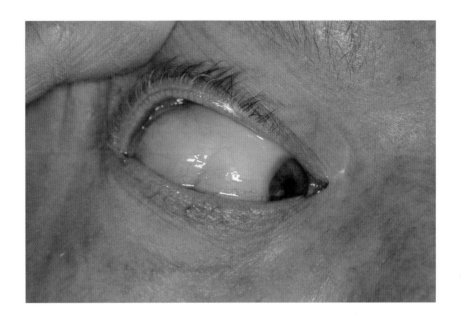

A 64-year-old man recently developed the mass evident in his right eye.

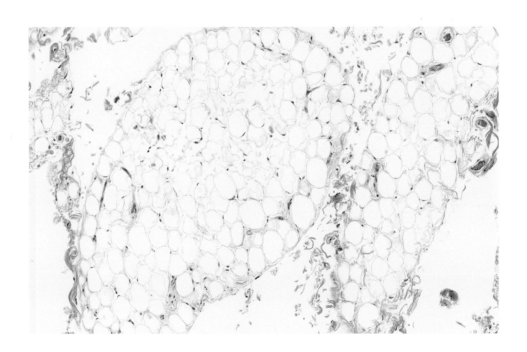

Diagnosis: Prolapsed orbital fat.

Clinical description: Clinical examination reveals prolapsed orbital fat.

Histological description: Histopathology demonstrates lobules of adipose tissue with intervening fibrovascular septae consistent with prolapsed orbital fat.

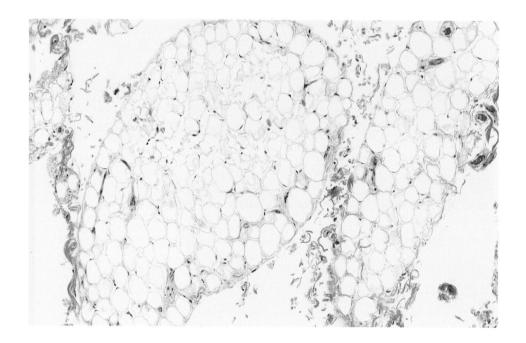

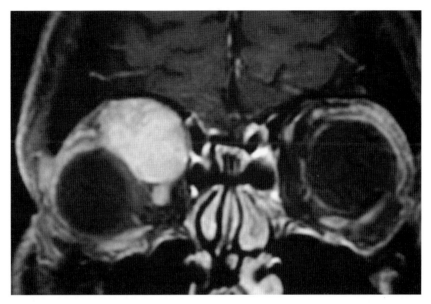

Courtesy of Jason A. Sokol, MD. Director of Oculofacial Plastic and Orbital Surgery at Kansas University Eye Center.

A 55-year-old man presented with diplopia for the past 6 months. The patient's CT scan is shown above.

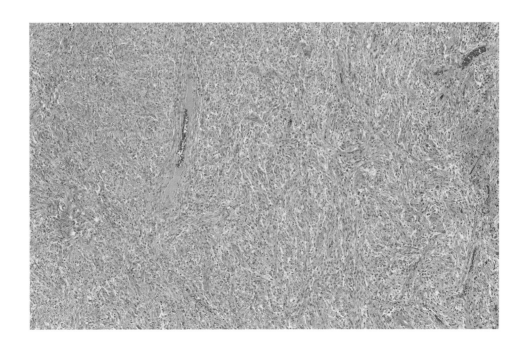

Diagnosis: Solitary fibrous tumor of the orbit.

Clinical description: T1-weighted magnetic resonance imaging demonstrates an enhancing, well-circumscribed lesion located superonasally in the right orbit.

Histological description: Sections through the specimen contain a very cellular connective tissue with spindle-shaped fibrocytes in a storiform pattern. Numerous fine vessels are seen coursing throughout the specimen. Larger slit-like vessels are also present (asterisks).

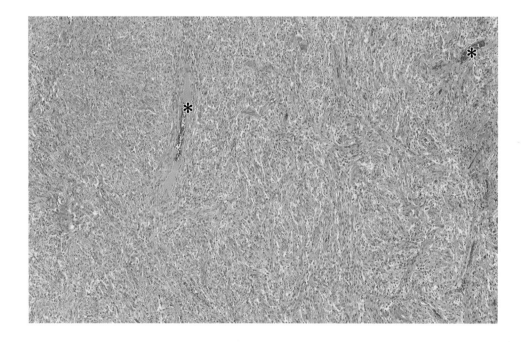

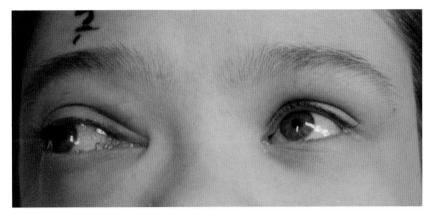

Courtesy of Jason A. Sokol, M.D. Director of Oculofacial Plastic and Orbital Surgery at Kansas University Eye Center.

A 10-year-old boy presented with a 2-month history of diplopia and exophthalmos of the right eye.

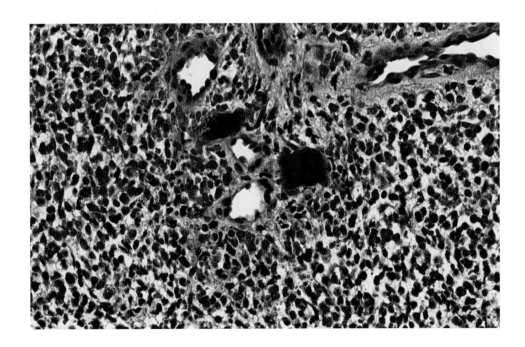

Diagnosis: Rhabdomyosarcoma.

Clinical description: Clinical examination reveals restriction of motility, mild proptosis, and right upper and lower eyelid fullness.

Histological description: Histopathological review of specimens using Masson trichrome reveals tissue composed of pleomorphic spindle-shaped cells with large, round dark nuclei. There are noted to be several areas where there are strap cells with markedly eosinophilic cytoplasm, the configuration of fibrils that reveal cross striations compatible with primitive skeletal muscle.

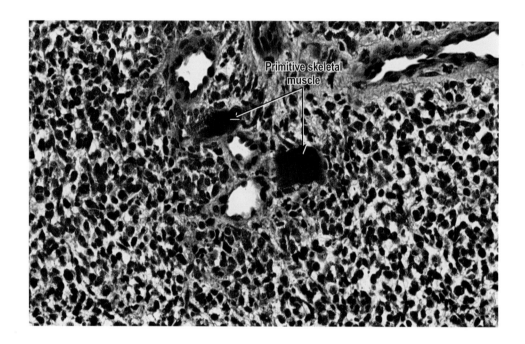

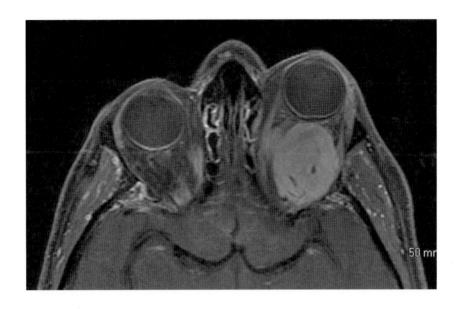

A 53-year-old patient presented with proptosis and double vision.

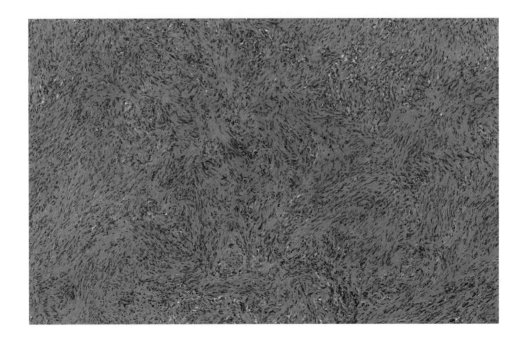

Diagnosis: Schwannoma.

Clinical description: T1-weighted magnetic resonance imaging shows a well-circumscribed intraconal mass in the left orbit.

Histological description: Section through the specimen shows scattered spindle-shaped cells growing in whorl pattern. There are areas of loosely and randomly spaced collagen bundles. S-100 stain is positive (not shown).

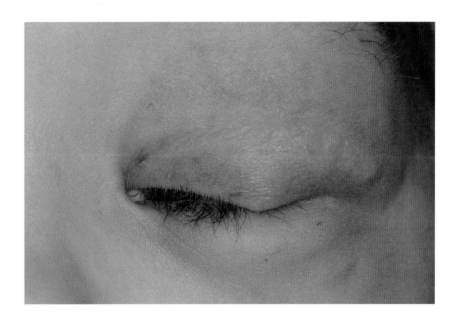

An 8-year-old boy presented with the above eyelid deformity.

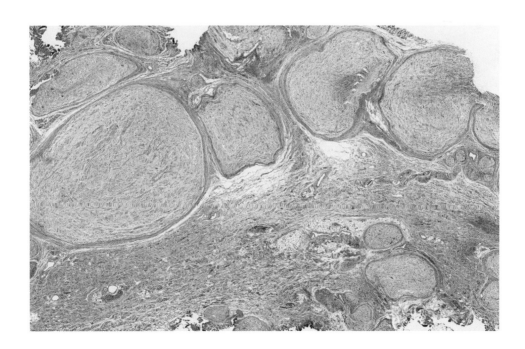

Diagnosis: Neurofibroma in a patient with neurofibromatosis.

Clinical description: The clinical examination reveals an "S-shaped" eyelid deformity.

Histological description: Histopathological evaluation shows multiple enlarged nerve bundles intertwined with collagen consistent with neurofibroma (asterisks).

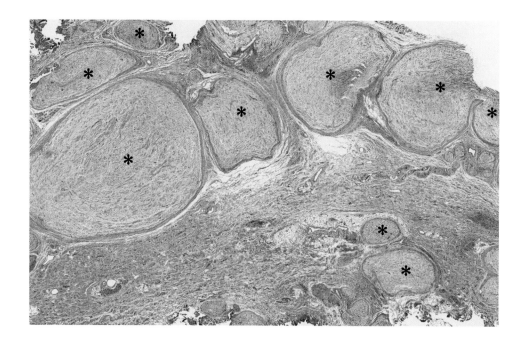

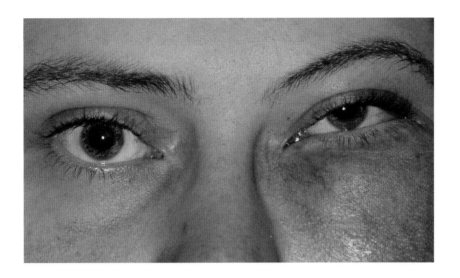

A 23-year-old man presented with diplopia and facial pain.

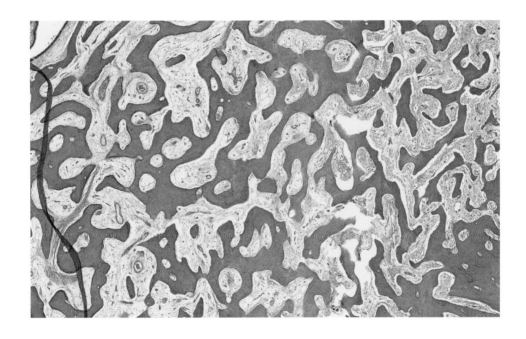

Diagnosis: Fibrous dysplasia.

Clinical description: Facial asymmetry with swelling of left side of the face is noted.

Histological description: Histopathological examination reveals irregular trabeculae of immature woven bone (resembling Chinese letters) in a fibrous background.

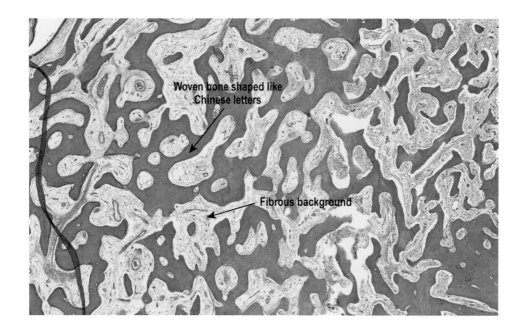

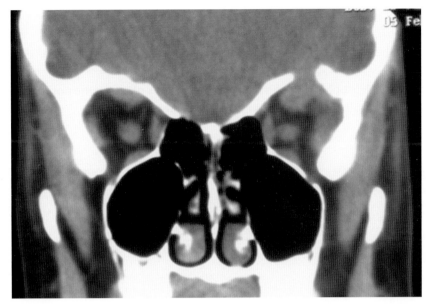

From Albert, Daniel M., Miller, Joan W., Azar, Dimitri T., and Blodi, Barbara A. (eds). 2008. Albert & Jakobiec's Principles and Practice of Ophthalmology, 3rd ed. Philadelphia: Copyright Elsevier 2008.

A 45-year-old patient presents with ocular pain and diplopia. The patient's CT scan is shown above.

Diagnosis: Eosinophilic granuloma.

Clinical description: The CT scan demonstrates a chronic lytic superior orbital lesion.

Histological description: Histopathology reveals two populations of cells. One population of cells is eosinophils (arrows) and the other population is epithelioid giant cells.

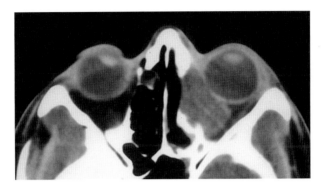

From Albert, Daniel M., Miller, Joan W., Azar, Dimitri T., and Blodi, Barbara A. (eds). 2008. Albert & Jakobiec's Principles and Practice of Ophthalmology, 3rd ed. Philadelphia: Copyright Elsevier 2008.

A 49-year-old female presented with eye pain and restricted ocular motility.

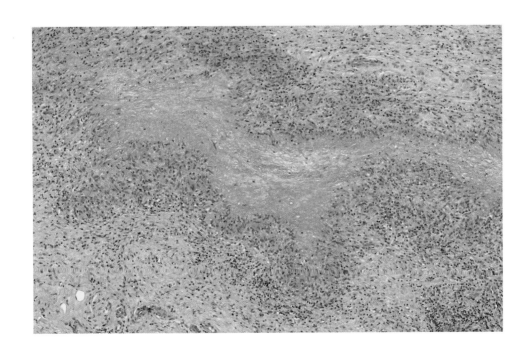

Diagnosis: Wegener's granulomatosis.

Clinical description: CT scan demonstrates a left orbital mass with erosion through the medial orbital wall. Patient tested positive for cANCA.

Histological description: Histopathology reveals areas of necrosis surrounded by epithelioid cells as well as lymphocytes, plasma cells, and a few neutrophils (asterisks).

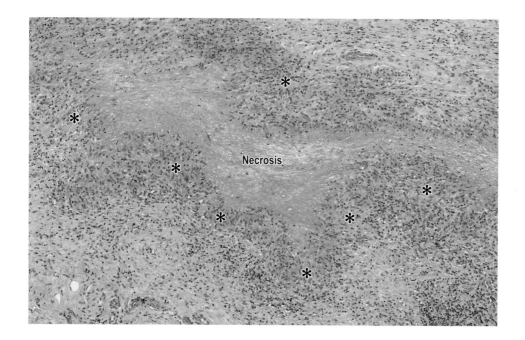

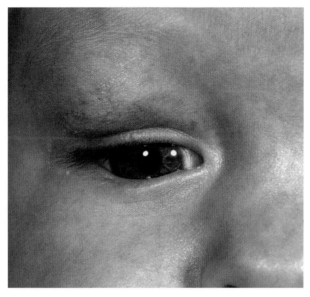

From Albert, Daniel M., Miller, Joan W., Azar, Dimitri T., and Blodi, Barbara A. (eds). 2008. Albert & Jakobiec's Principles and Practice of Ophthalmology, 3rd ed. Philadelphia: Copyright Elsevier 2008.

A 1-year-old child presented with ptosis and a right superior orbital mass, depicted above. He underwent an orbital biopsy.

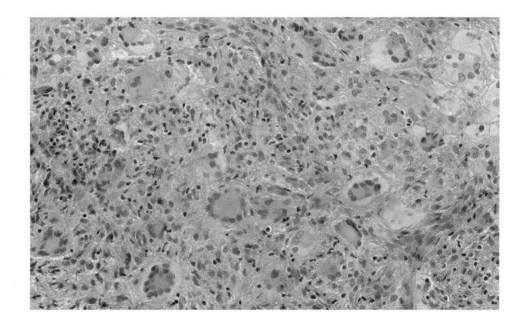

Diagnosis: Juvenile xanthogranuloma with primary orbital involvement.

Clinical description: Clinical examination reveals a right upper eyelid swelling causing ptosis in this 1-year-old patient.

Histological description: Orbital biopsy reveals a histiocytic cell tumor containing numerous Touton multinucleated giant cells (arrows).

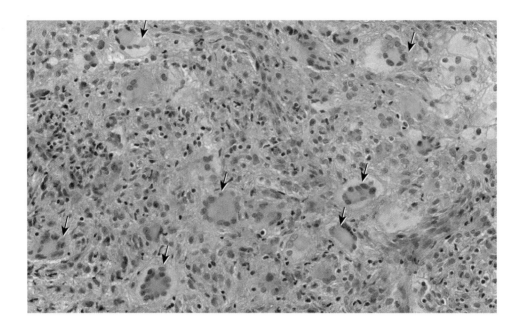

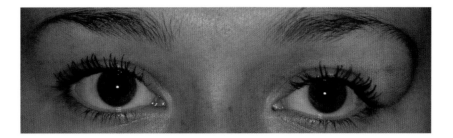

A 19-year-old woman presented with a 4-month history of left upper eyelid fullness. She underwent anterior orbitotomy.

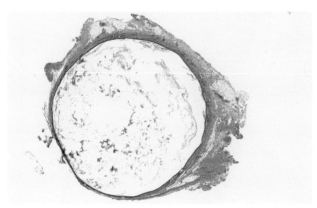 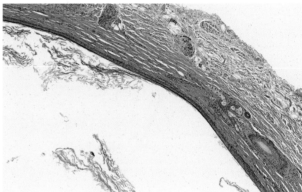

Diagnosis: Dermoid cyst.

Clinical description: Left upper eyelid swelling and fullness is noted temporally.

Histological description: A large cystic cavity filled with keratin is seen (top). Higher magnification (bottom) shows that the cystic cavity is lined by keratinized stratified squamous epithelium and associated pilosebaceous units.

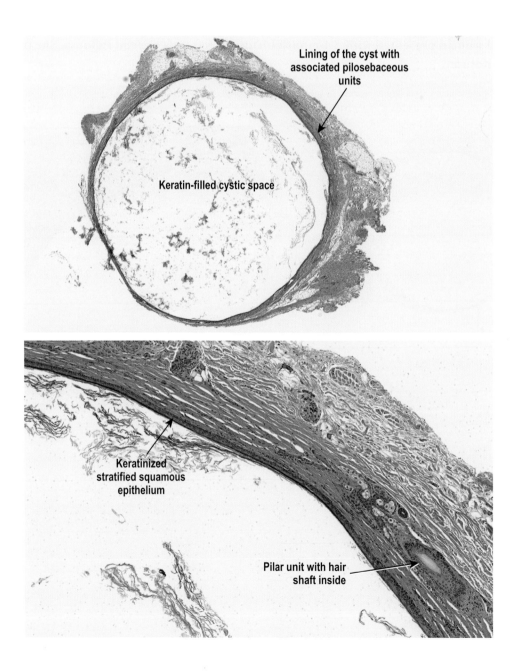

Lining of the cyst with associated pilosebaceous units

Keratin-filled cystic space

Keratinized stratified squamous epithelium

Pilar unit with hair shaft inside

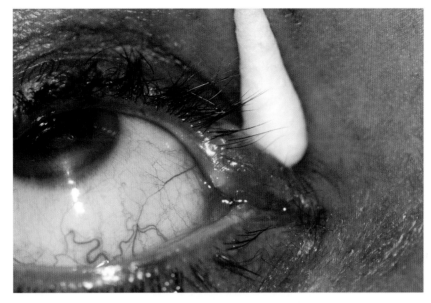

Courtesy of Jason A. Sokol, MD. Director of Oculofacial Plastic and Orbital Surgery at Kansas University Eye Center.

A 36-year-old woman presented with pain, redness, and swelling of her right upper eyelid. The material in the upper canaliculi was expressed and examined microscopically.

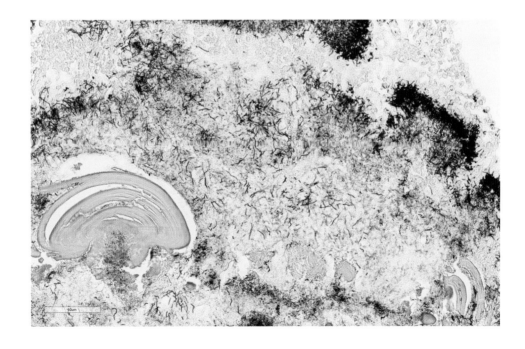

Diagnosis: Canaliculitis secondary to *Actinomyces*.

Clinical description: Granular calcified material is being expressed from the upper punctum.

Histological description: Clusters of Gram-positive filaments are seen in a matrix of calcified mineralized tissue.

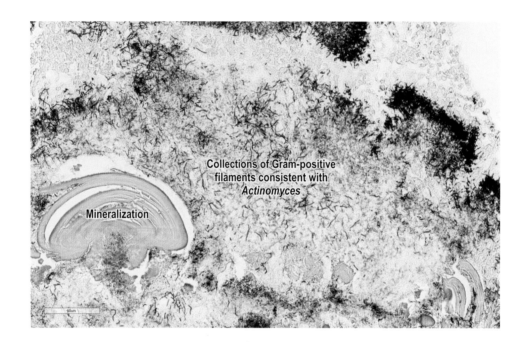

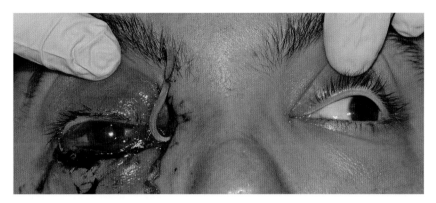

Courtesy of Jason A. Sokol, MD. Director of Oculofacial Plastic and Orbital Surgery at Kansas University Eye Center.

A 27-year-old diabetic man presented with right eyelid swelling and a frozen globe.

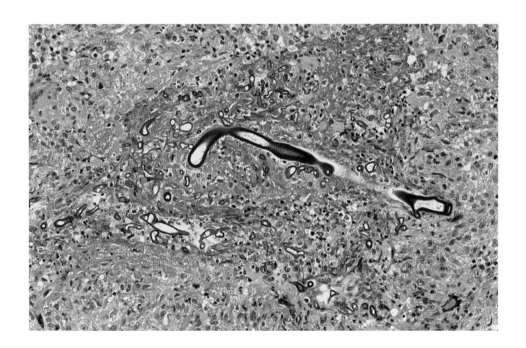

Diagnosis: Orbital infection with mucormycosis.

Clinical description: Swelling of the upper and lower eyelids with pigmented discharge is noted on clinical examination.

Histological description: Nonseptate filamentous fungi consistent with Mucor are seen (arrows).

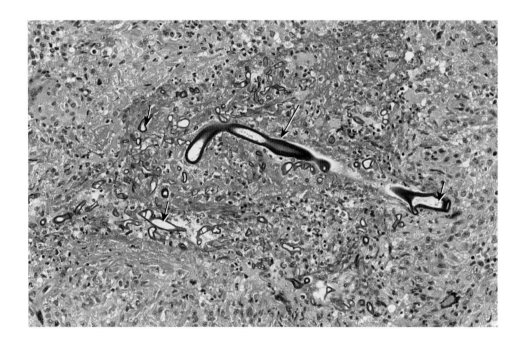

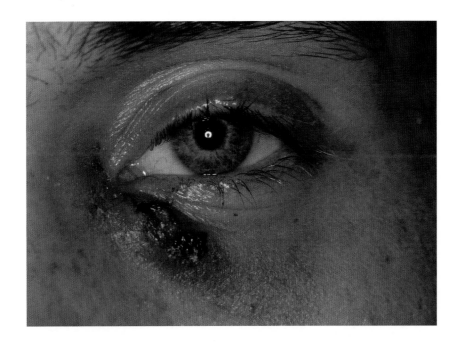

A 37-year-old man presented with epiphora, swelling, and pain in the left medial canthus area. He underwent a dacryocystorhinostomy.

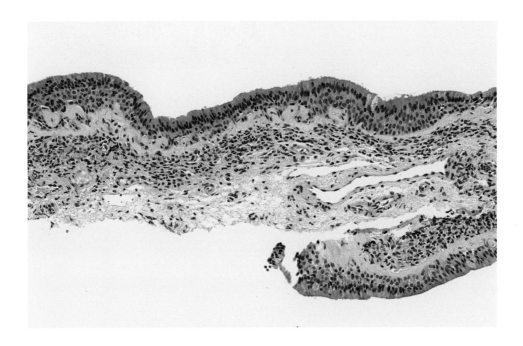

Diagnosis: Dacryocystitis.

Clinical description: Clinical examination revealed redness and swelling along the left medial canthus. The overlying skin is ulcerated.

Histological description: Histopathology reveals tissue lined by nonkeratinized, pseudostratified columnar epithelium with mucus glands. Chronic nongranulomatous inflammation consisting of lymphocytes and plasma cells is seen infiltrating the stroma (arrowheads). Gram stain reveals small clusters of Gram-positive cocci (not shown).

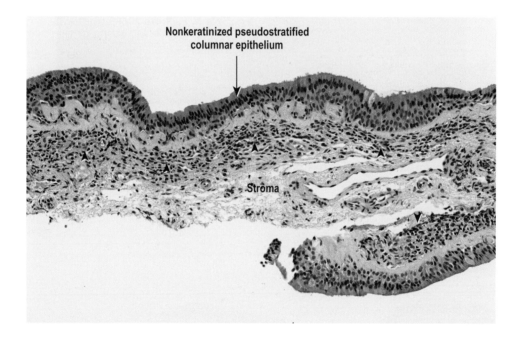

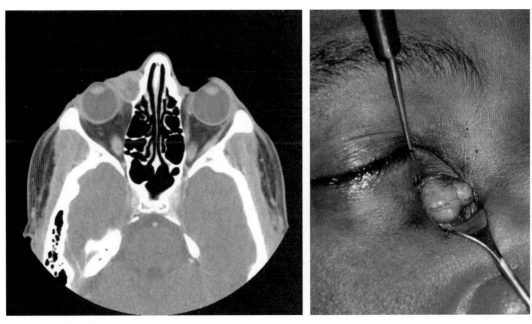

Printed with permission from Azari A.A., Kanavi M.R., Saipe N., Lee V., Lucarelli M., Potter H.D., Albert D.M. Transitional Cell Carcinoma of the Lacrimal Sac Presenting With Bloody Tears. JAMA Ophthalmology 2013; 131(5):689–690.

A 54-year-old man presented with swelling of the right lower eyelid and bloody tears for the past 6 months.

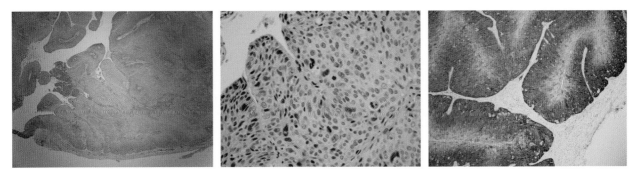

Printed with permission from Azari A.A., Kanavi M.R., Saipe N., Lee V., Lucarelli M., Potter H.D., Albert D.M. Transitional Cell Carcinoma of the Lacrimal Sac Presenting With Bloody Tears. JAMA Ophthalmology 2013; 131(5):689–690.

Diagnosis: Transitional cell carcinoma of the lacrimal sac.

Clinical description: The CT scan shows a heterogeneous, well-circumscribed mass in the right lacrimal sac fossa. Intraoperative photograph reveals a large mass within the lacrimal sac.

Histological description: Histopathological examination reveals papillary proliferation of transitional cells (left). Nuclear pleomorphism and few mitotic figures are noted (center). Immunohistochemistry for HPV-16 is diffusely positive, suggesting HPV involvement (right).

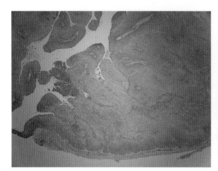 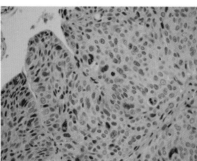 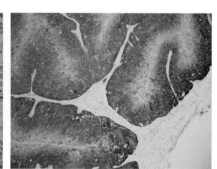

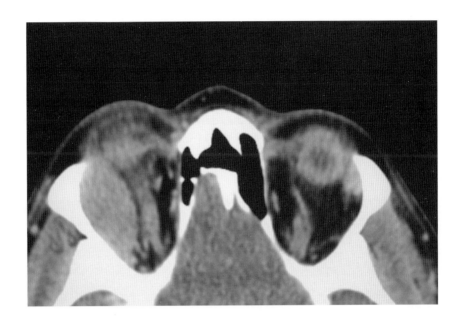

A 58-year-old man presented with a 6-month history of double vision. He later underwent an orbital biopsy.

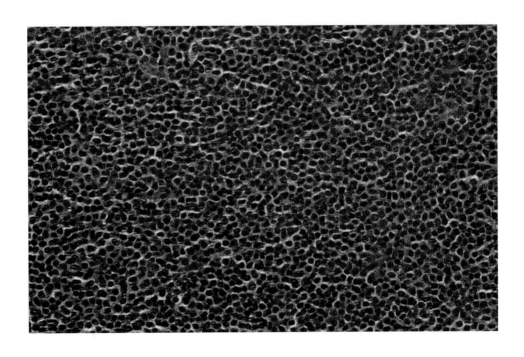

Diagnosis: Orbital lymphoma (small B-lymphocytic lymphoma).

Clinical description: CT scan shows infiltration of the right orbit. The tumor appears to be conforming to the lateral orbital wall.

Histological description: Histopathology demonstrates dense infiltrate of small, round, uniform, basophilic cells. Immunohistochemistry was strongly positive for CD20 (not shown).

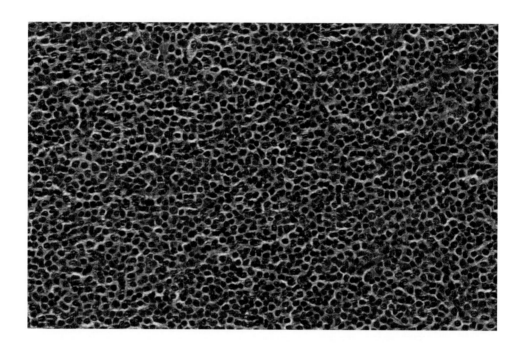

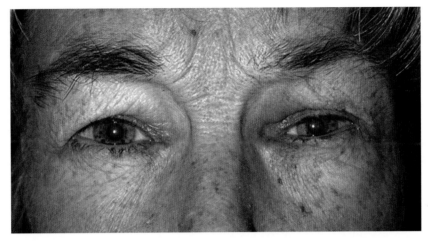

From Albert, Daniel M., Miller, Joan W., Azar, Dimitri T., and Blodi, Barbara A. (eds). 2008. Albert & Jakobiec's Principles and Practice of Ophthalmology, 3rd ed. Philadelphia: Copyright Elsevier 2008.

An 85-year-old woman with a history of breast cancer presented with diplopia and a "smaller left eye."

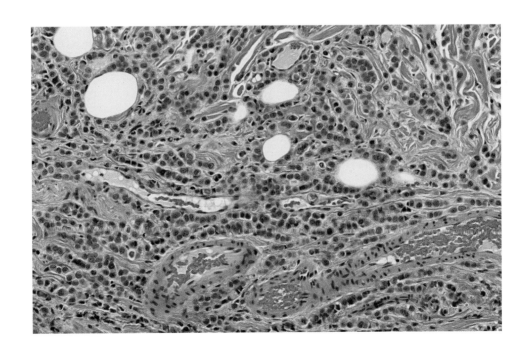

Diagnosis: Breast cancer with orbital cancer.

Clinical description: Clinical examination demonstrates left eye enophthalmos and narrowing of the palpebral fissure.

Histological description: Histopathology reveals tissue infiltrated with epithelial cells in an "Indian-file" arrangement (arrows). These cells are round with eosinophilic cytoplasm and round to irregular nuclei displaying moderate atypia, including pleomorphism, an enlarged nucleus-to-cytoplasm ratio, and prominent nucleoli. There are occasional areas of duct formation (asterisks).

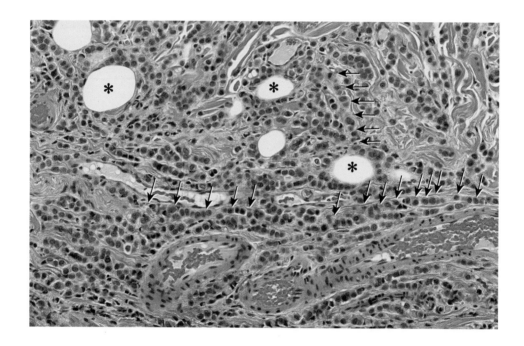

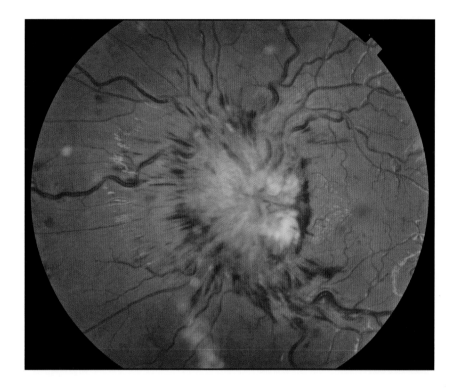

A 37-year-old obese woman presented with decreased vision and chronic headaches.

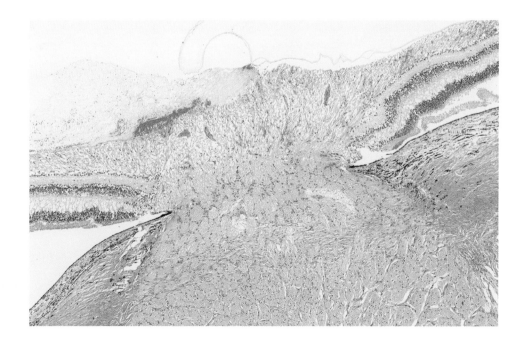

Diagnosis: Papilledema due to idiopathic intracranial hypertension.

Clinical description: Dilated fundus examination shows swelling of the optic nerve head surrounded by hemorrhages.

Histological description: Histopathology demonstrates swelling and anterior displacement of the optic nerve head.

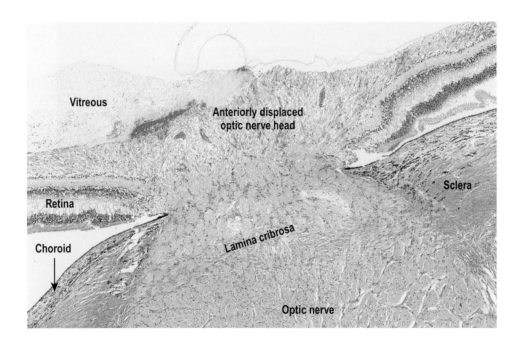

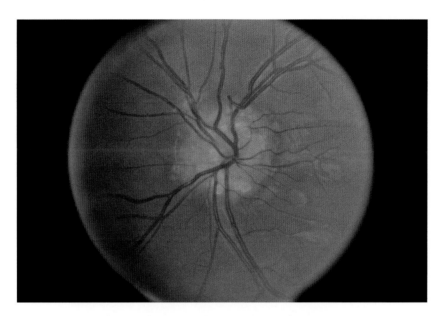

A 29-year-old man was referred for evaluation of optic nerve edema.

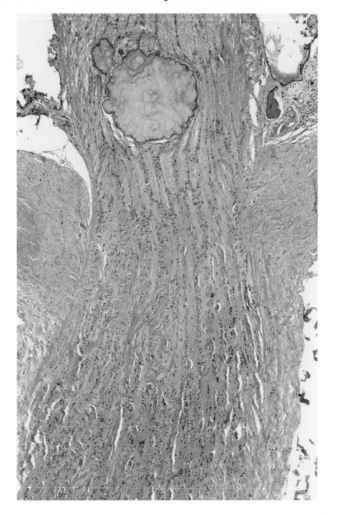

Diagnosis: Optic nerve drusen.

Clinical description: Close inspection of the optic nerve head reveals deposition of hyaline material within the optic nerve head.

Histological description: Calcified deposits are seen within the optic nerve head anterior to the lamina cribrosa.

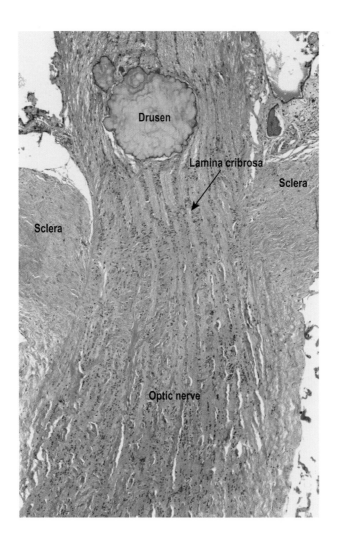

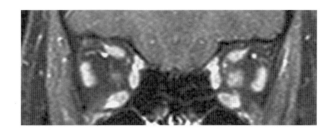

A 32-year-old woman presented with a sudden onset of decreased vision and the above MRI findings.

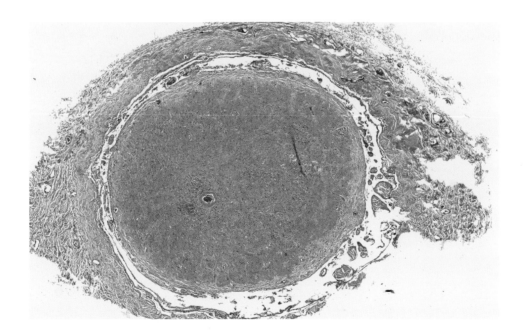

Diagnosis: Optic neuritis.

Clinical description: Magnetic resonance imaging demonstrates enhancement of the left optic nerve consistent with optic neuritis.

Histological description: Histopathology demonstrates a cross-sectional view of the optic nerve. An area of lymphoplasmacytic inflammation is seen within the optic nerve near a central retinal vessel.

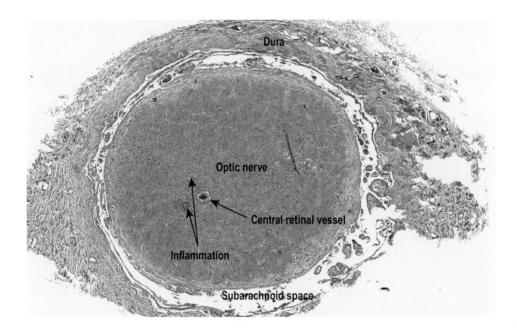

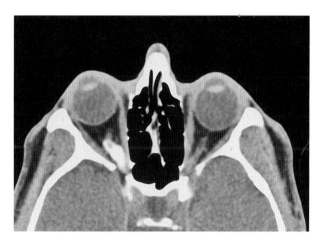

From Albert, Daniel M., Miller, Joan W., Azar, Dimitri T., and Blodi, Barbara A. (eds). 2008. Albert & Jakobiec's Principles and Practice of Ophthalmology, 3rd ed. Philadelphia: Copyright Elsevier 2008.

A 47-year-old woman presented with mild blurring of the vision in her right eye.

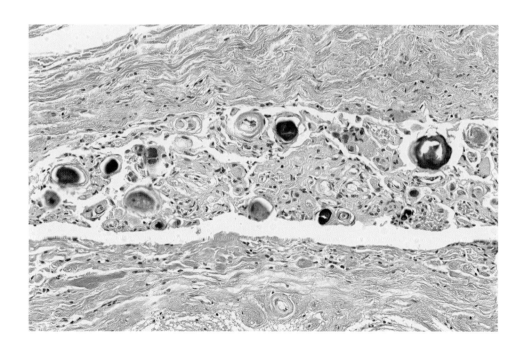

Diagnosis: Optic nerve sheath meningioma.

Clinical description: Axial CT scan imaging shows calcification of the optic nerve posteriorly and the classic "tram-tracking" appearance anteriorly.

Histological description: Histopathology demonstrates proliferation of meningothelial cells surrounding the optic nerve. Many calcified psammoma bodies are present (asterisks).

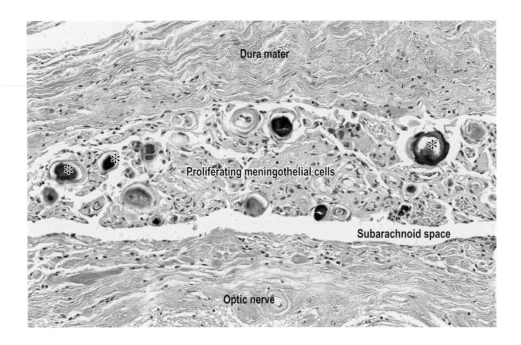

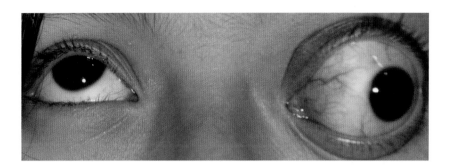

A 14-year-old girl presented with progressive proptosis over the past 9 months.

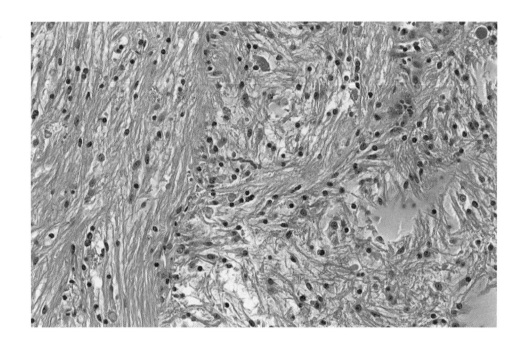

Diagnosis: Optic nerve glioma.

Clinical description: Left eye proptosis and restricted extraocular motility is noted.

Histological description: The tumor demonstrates proliferation of pilocytic glial cells and astrocytes (arrowhead). Rosenthal fibers (eosinophilic bundles of fibrils), which are pathognomonic for this condition are seen.

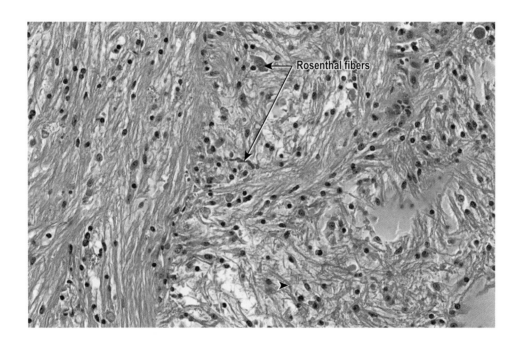

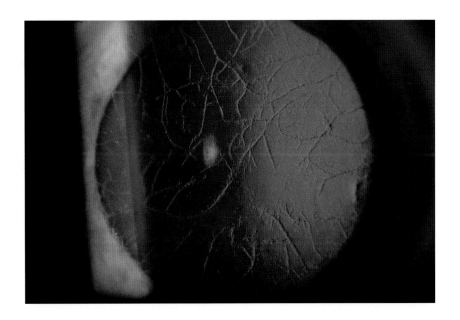

A 41-year-old woman presented with a longstanding history of corneal findings, as shown above.

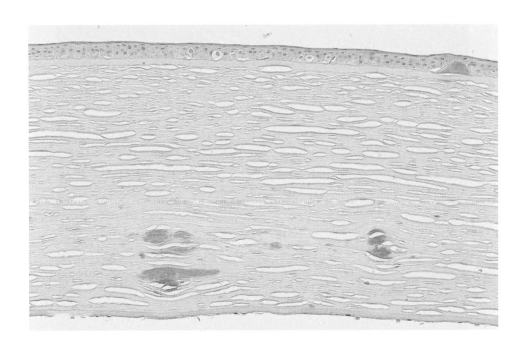

Diagnosis: Lattice dystrophy.

Clinical description: The slit-lamp exam demonstrates linear bands of corneal opacification.

Histological description: Histopathology reveals amorphous deposits that stain positive with Congo red (previous page) and show birefringence (green and orange) under the polarized light.

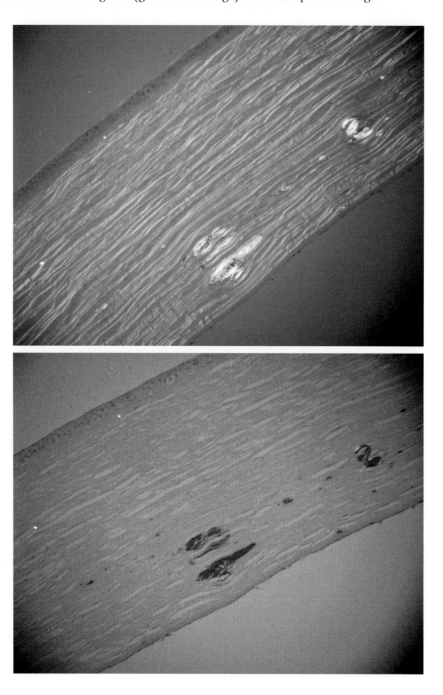

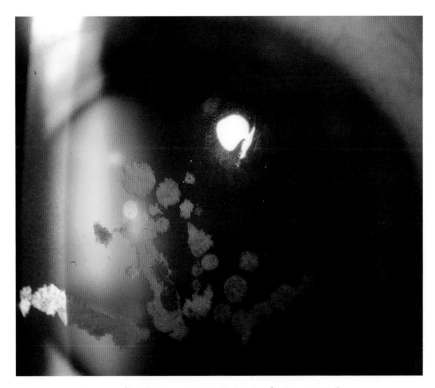

Courtesy of Neal P. Barney, M.D. University of Wisconsin-Madison.

A 23-year-old man presented with corneal opacities, as shown above. He later underwent a penetrating keratoplasty.

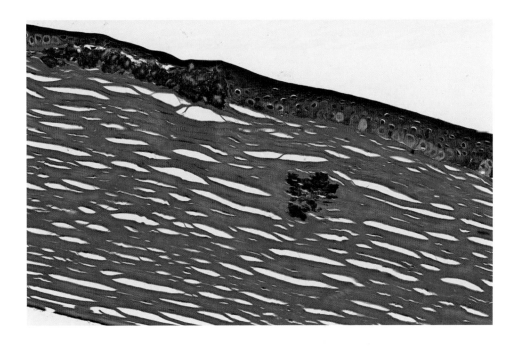

Diagnosis: Granular dystrophy.

Clinical description: Anterior stromal opacities are seen with clear intervening spaces. The corneal opacity does not involve the peripheral cornea.

Histological description: Staining with Masson trichrome demonstrates subepithelial as well as anterior stromal corneal infiltrates (arrows). The deposits are composed of hyaline and stain red with Masson trichrome.

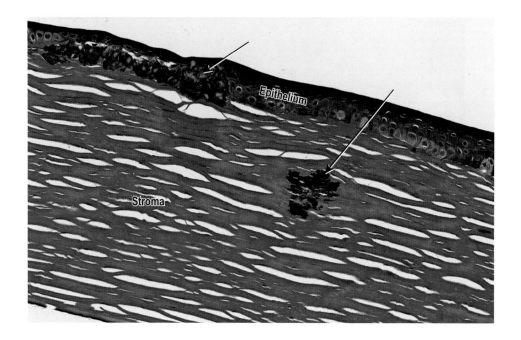

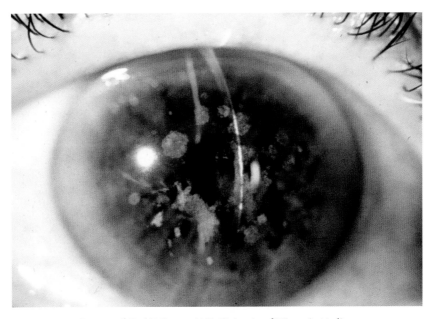

Courtesy of Neal P. Barney, M.D. University of Wisconsin-Madison.

A 32-year-old woman presented with decreased vision. She later underwent penetrating keratoplasty.

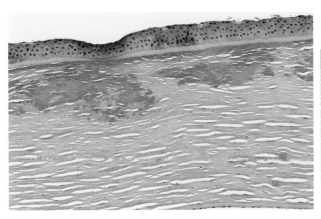 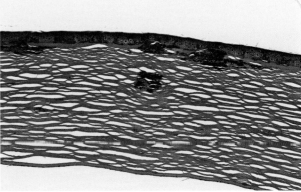

Diagnosis: Avellino corneal dystrophy.

Clinical description: Slit-lamp examination reveals multiple confluent well-circumscribed stromal opacities.

Histological description: The histopathology has features of both lattice and granular dystrophy. PAS stain deposits (arrow, top) that also stain positive with Congo red and demonstrate dichroism under the polarized light (not shown), typical of lattice dystrophy. Masson trichrome staining shows hyaline deposits in the anterior stroma, as seen in granular dystrophy (bottom). Hyaline deposits are shown with arrows.

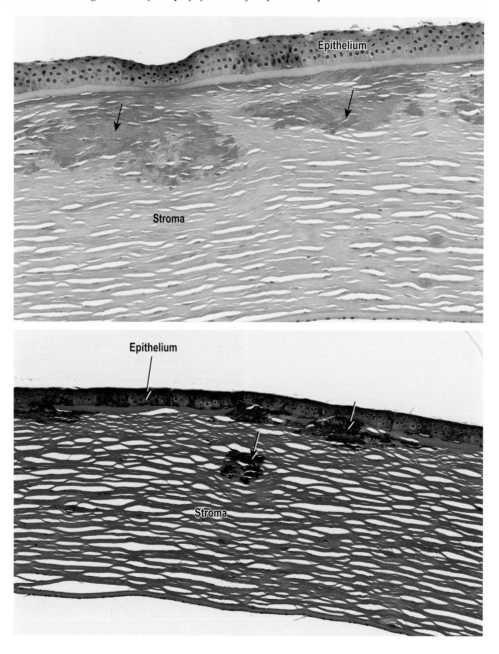

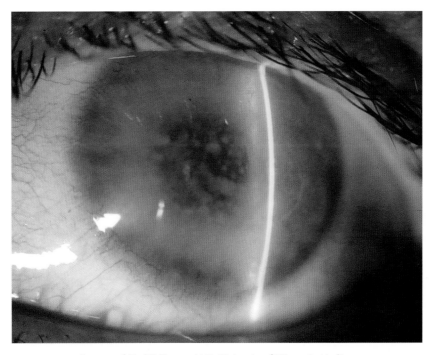

Courtesy of Neal P. Barney, M.D. University of Wisconsin-Madison.

A 19-year-old patient presented with decreased vision and photophobia.

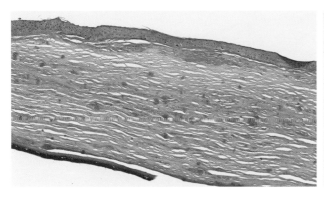 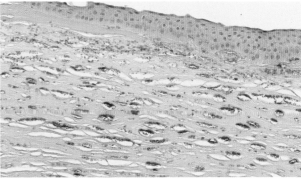

Diagnosis: Macular dystrophy.

Clinical description: Confluent corneal opacities extending to the limbus without clear intervening spaces are seen on the slit-lamp examination.

Histological description: Infiltrates are seen at all levels. Alcian blue demonstrates positive staining of the mucopolysaccharide deposits.

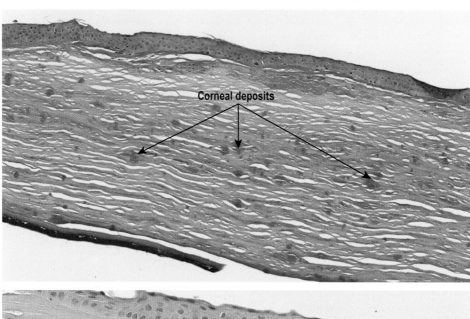

Corneal deposits

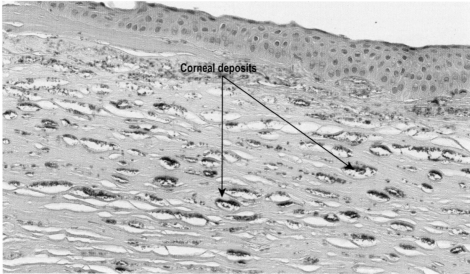

Corneal deposits

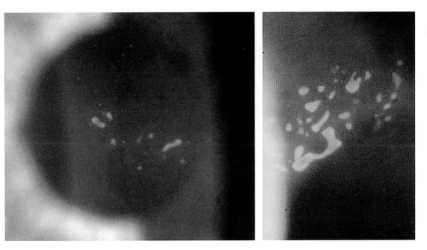

From Albert, Daniel M., Miller, Joan W., Azar, Dimitri T., and Blodi, Barbara A. (eds). 2008. Albert & Jakobiec's Principles and Practice of Ophthalmology, 3rd ed. Philadelphia: Copyright Elsevier 2008.

A 38-year-old woman with a history of ocular pain, and foreign body sensation, worse in the morning, presented with the above slit-lamp examination finding.

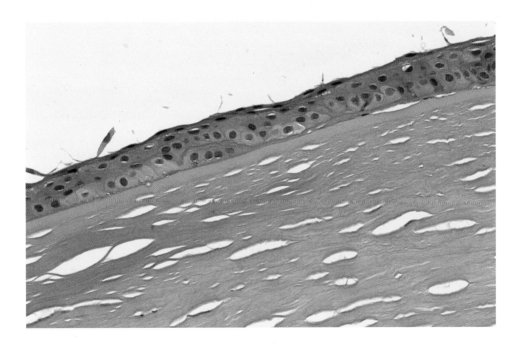

Diagnosis: Anterior basement membrane dystrophy.

Clinical description: The slit-lamp examination demonstrates the typical "map" dystrophy within the anterior cornea.

Histological description: Histopathology demonstrates reduplicated epithelial basement membrane. There is also separation of the epithelial basement membrane from the underlying Bowman's layer in some areas (arrowhead).

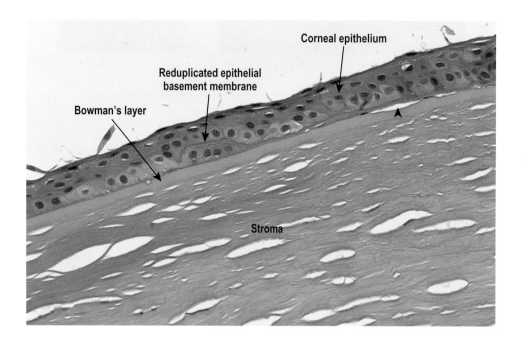

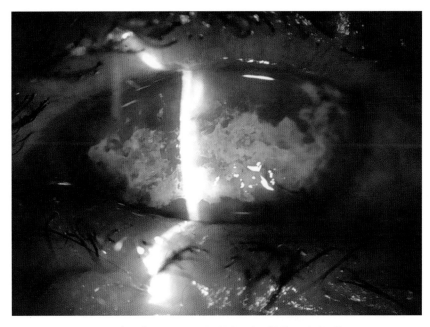

Courtesy of Neal P. Barney, M.D. University of Wisconsin-Madison.

A 56-year-old patient with a past ocular history of longstanding retinal detachment presented with decreased vision and ocular pain.

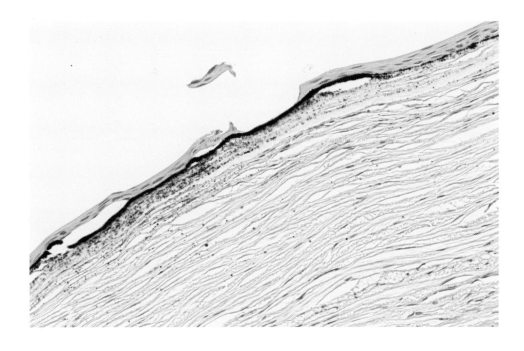

Diagnosis: Band keratopathy.

Clinical description: Cornea is deposited with plaques of calcified material.

Histological description: von Kossa stain demonstrates calcium deposits within the epithelial basement membrane and Bowman's layer. The surface epithelium is attenuated and absent in some areas.

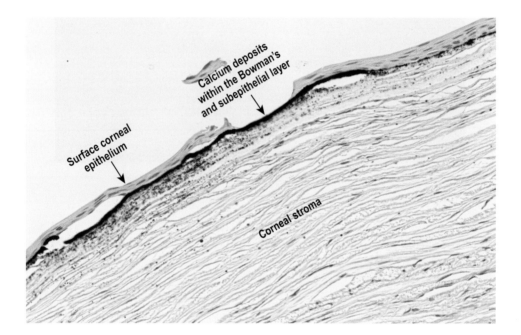

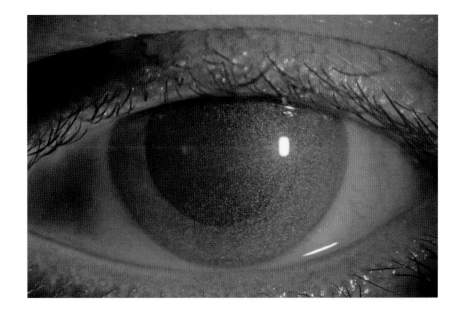

A 6-year-old patient with bilateral corneal opacity underwent penetrating keratoplasty and conjunctival biopsy.

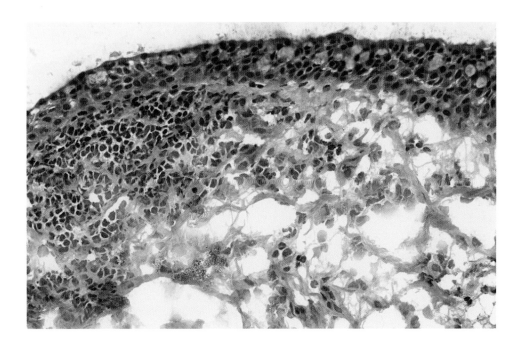

Diagnosis: Cystinosis.

Clinical description: Clinical examination reveals punctate areas of opacity within the corneal stroma.

Histological description: Histopathology reveals goblet cells containing nonkeratinized stratified squamous epithelium. Cystine crystals (circles) are seen within the conjunctival stroma.

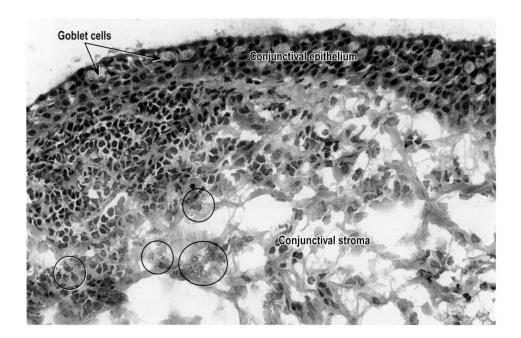

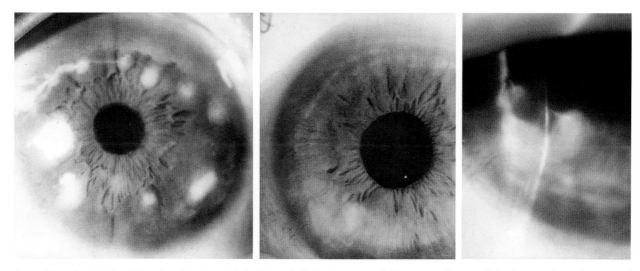

From Albert, Daniel M., Miller, Joan W., Azar, Dimitri T., and Blodi, Barbara A. (eds). 2008. Albert & Jakobiec's Principles and Practice of Ophthalmology, 3rd ed. Philadelphia: Copyright Elsevier 2008.

A 43-year-old patient presented with dry eyes and foreign body sensation.

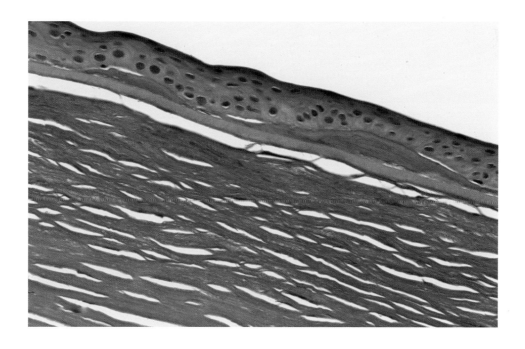

Diagnosis: Salzmann's nodular degeneration.

Clinical description: The slit-lamp examination reveals multiple bluish-gray elevated anterior corneal nodules.

Histological description: Examination of the histopathological sections reveals thick, fibrous tissue (asterisks) interposed between Bowman's membrane and the irregular epithelium.

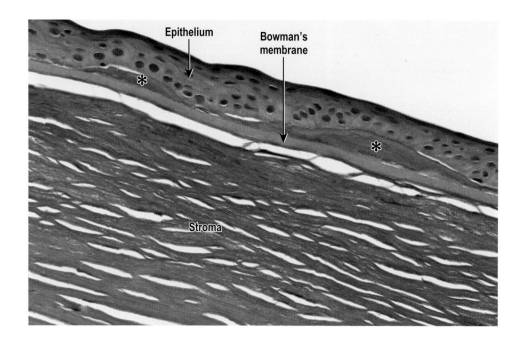

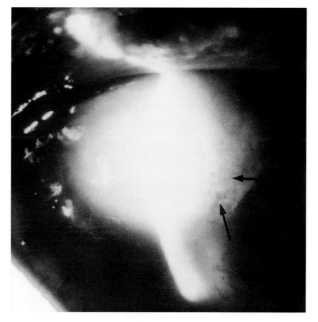

From Albert, Daniel M., Miller, Joan W., Azar, Dimitri T., and Blodi, Barbara A. (eds). 2008. Albert & Jakobiec's Principles and Practice of Ophthalmology, 3rd ed. Philadelphia: Copyright Elsevier 2008.

A 53-year-old man presented with bilateral decreased vision with the above external appearance. He had similar findings in his other eye.

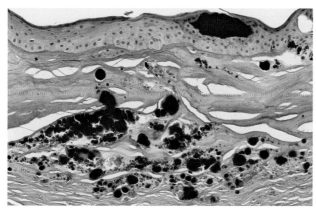
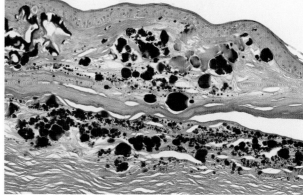

Diagnosis: Spheroidal degeneration.

Clinical description: The slit-lamp photograph demonstrates many spheroidal deposits within the stroma of the cornea.

Histological description: Sections through the specimen show amorphous deposits of varying size in the anterior stroma and epithelium (arrows) that are markedly positive with elastin stain (bottom). Extensive subepithelial fibrosis is seen. The epithelium is of variable thickness and shows intracellular edema.

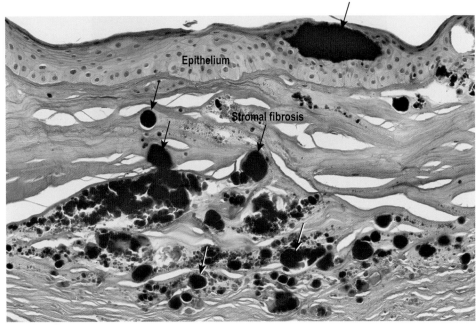

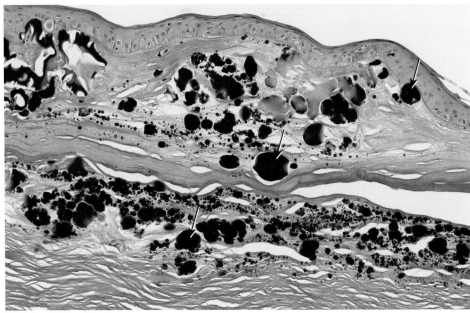

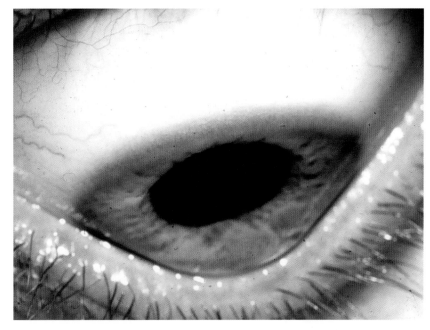

Courtesy of Neal P. Barney, M.D. University of Wisconsin-Madison.

A 25-year-old man presented with decreased vision and the above ophthalmic examination finding.

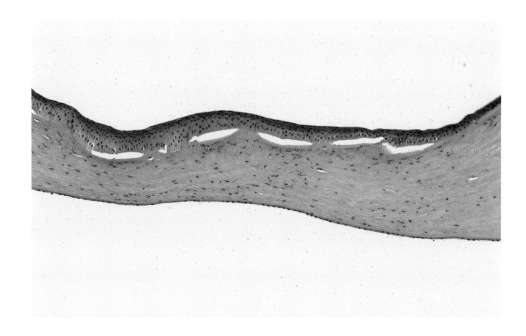

Diagnosis: Keratoconus.

Clinical description: Cone-shape deformity of the cornea along with the classic Munson's sign (V-shaped deformity of the lower eyelid in downward gaze) is demonstrated.

Histological description: Histopathology demonstrates a thinned cornea with attenuated epithelium. Multiple breaks (arrowheads) within the Bowman's layer are seen. The endothelium is well preserved.

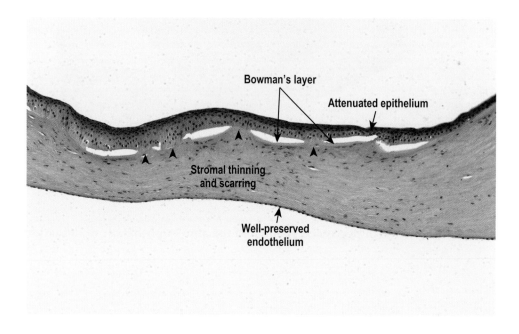

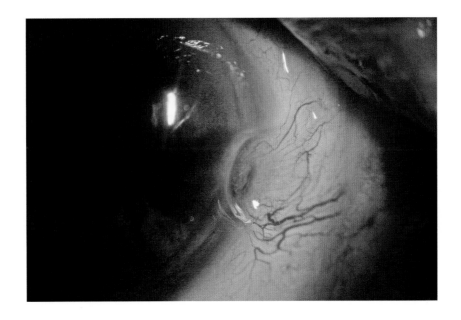

A 72-year-old man presented with dry eyes and the above clinical picture.

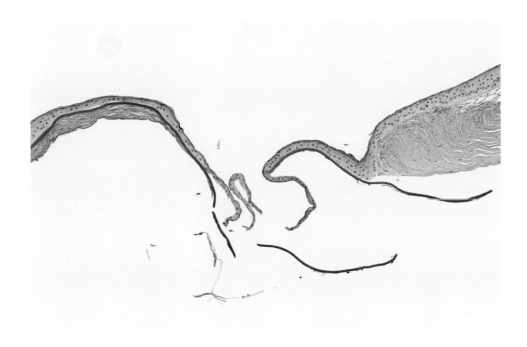

Diagnosis: Corneal dellen.

Clinical description: Slit-lamp examination reveals corneal thinning just inside the limbus.

Histological description: Histopathology reveals corneal thinning with artifactuous breaks in the Descemet's membrane.

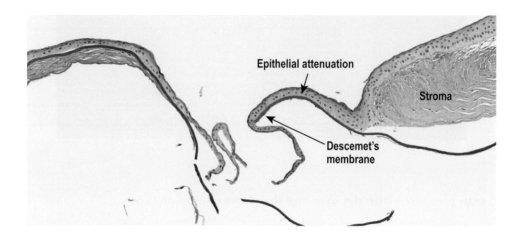

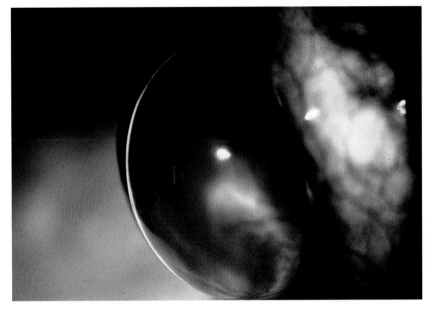

Courtesy of Neal P. Barney, M.D. University of Wisconsin-Madison.

A 55-year-old man presented with poor vision, which could not be improved with refraction.

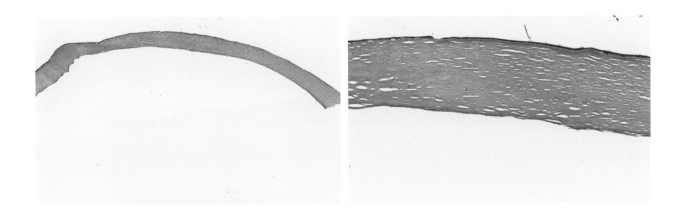

Diagnosis: Keratoglobus.

Clinical description: The slit-lamp examination shows generalized thinning and globular protrusion of the cornea.

Histological description: The cornea is thin centrally as well as peripherally. The epithelium is attenuated with loss of Bowman's layer in some areas.

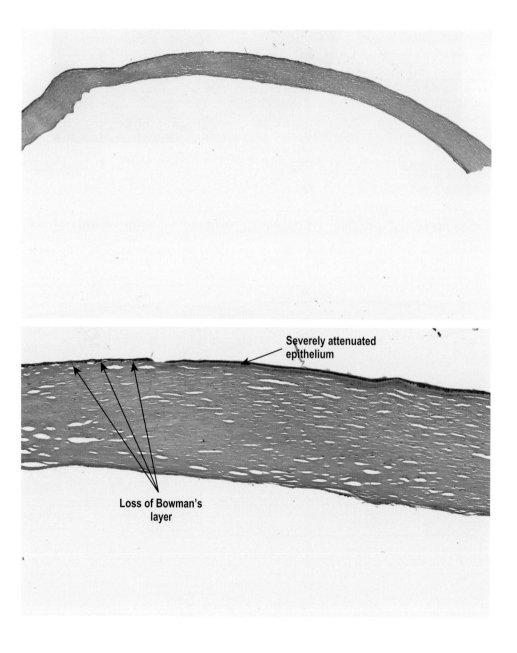

Severely attenuated epithelium

Loss of Bowman's layer

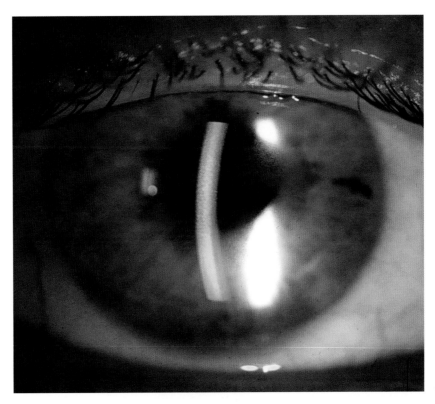

Courtesy of Neal P. Barney, M.D. University of Wisconsin-Madison.

A 69-year-old woman presented with decreased vision, worse upon waking up. After failing medical therapy, she underwent a penetrating keratoplasty.

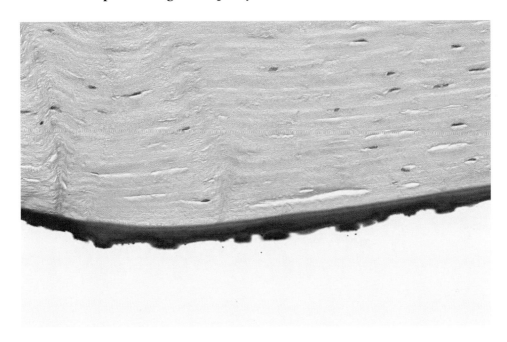

Diagnosis: Fuchs' endothelial dystrophy.

Clinical description: Slit-lamp examination reveals marked corneal edema with a "beaten bronze" appearance to the posterior cornea.

Histological description: An edematous cornea with loss of normal stromal cleft is seen. Anvil-shaped excrescences consistent with guttae are seen.

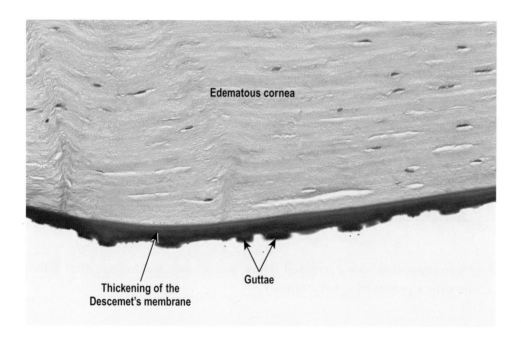

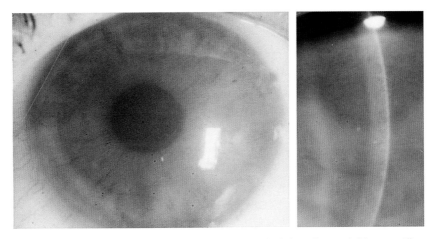

From Albert, Daniel M., Miller, Joan W., Azar, Dimitri T., and Blodi, Barbara A. (eds). 2008. Albert & Jakobiec's Principles and Practice of Ophthalmology, 3rd ed. Philadelphia: Copyright Elsevier 2008.

A 16-month-old infant presented with decreased vision and nystagmus.

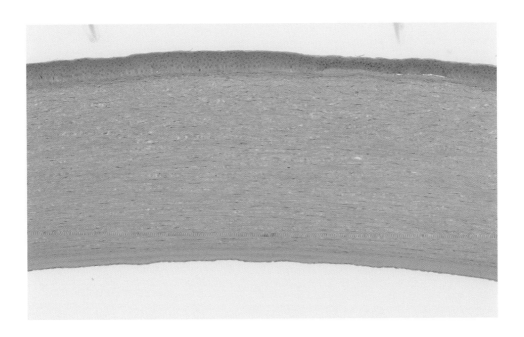

Diagnosis: Congenital hereditary endothelial dystrophy (CHED).

Clinical description: Slit-lamp examination reveals mild corneal haze.

Histological description: Histopathology reveals a thickened cornea with loss of natural stromal clefts. The Descemet's membrane is thick and the endothelial cell layer is absent.

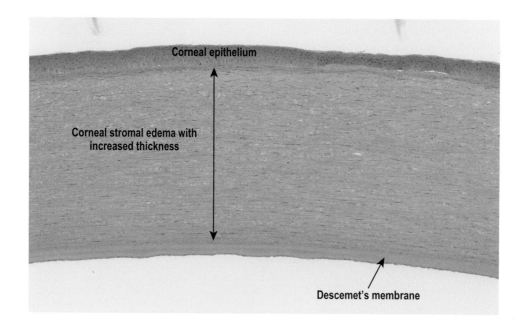

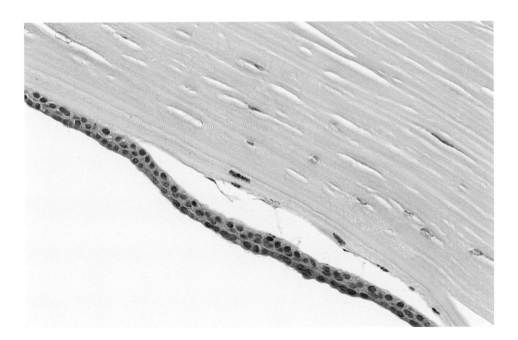

Courtesy of Neal P. Barney, M.D. University of Wisconsin-Madison.

A 4-year-old girl with decreased vision since birth presented with the above corneal finding on slit-lamp examination. She later underwent a penetrating keratoplasty.

Diagnosis: Posterior polymorphous dystrophy.

Clinical description: Slit-lamp examination reveals multiple scalloped corneal opacities located posteriorly.

Histological description: Histopathology demonstrates a multilayer endothelium.

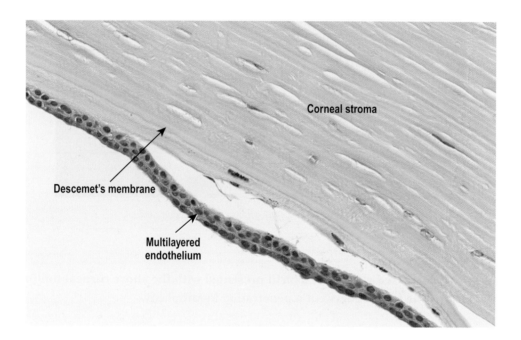

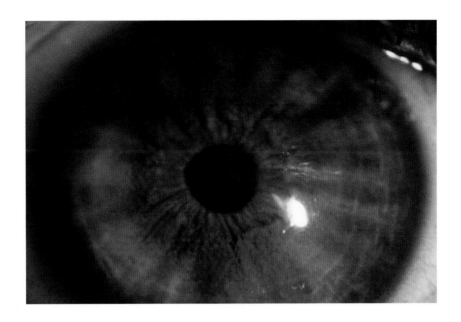

A 32-year-old man with no ocular complaints presented for a routine eye examination.

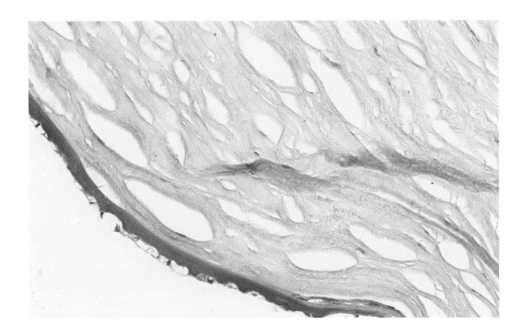

Diagnosis: Hassall–Henle bodies.

Clinical description: A slit-lamp examination reveals a normal cornea.

Histological description: Histopathology demonstrates peripheral guttae in this otherwise normal cornea.

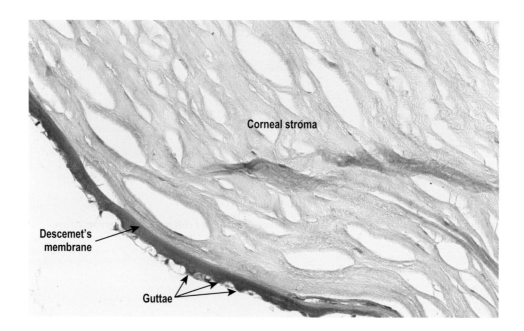

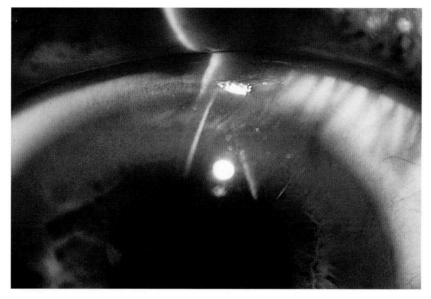

From Albert, Daniel M., Miller, Joan W., Azar, Dimitri T., and Blodi, Barbara A. (eds). 2008. Albert & Jakobiec's Principles and Practice of Ophthalmology, 3rd ed. Philadelphia: Copyright Elsevier 2008.

A 77-year-old terminally ill patient was seen as an inpatient with the above slit-lamp examination finding.

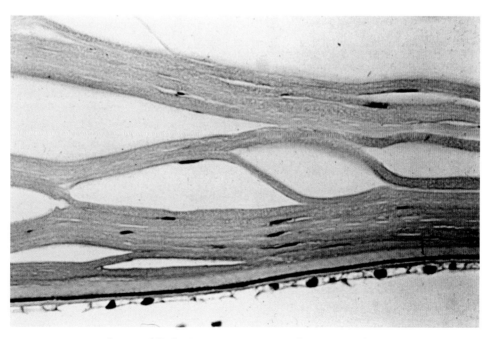

Courtesy of Neal P. Barney, M.D. University of Wisconsin-Madison.

Diagnosis: Wilson's disease.

Clinical description: Slit-lamp examination reveals a pigmented Descemet's membrane consistent with Kayser–Fleischer ring.

Histological description: Histopathology demonstrates a dark band of copper deposit on the posterior aspect of the Descemet's membrane (short arrows).

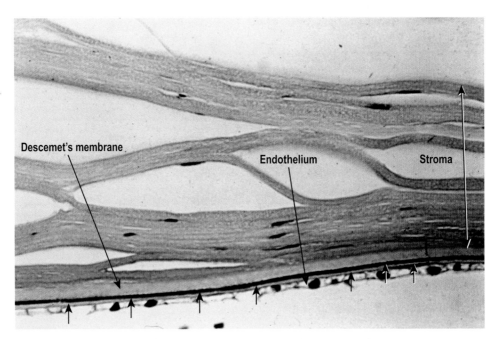

Courtesy of Neal P. Barney, M.D. University of Wisconsin-Madison.

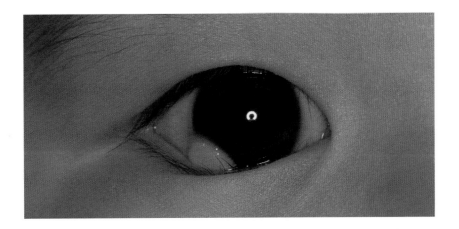

A 2-year-old boy with a history of Goldenhar syndrome presented with a limbal mass.

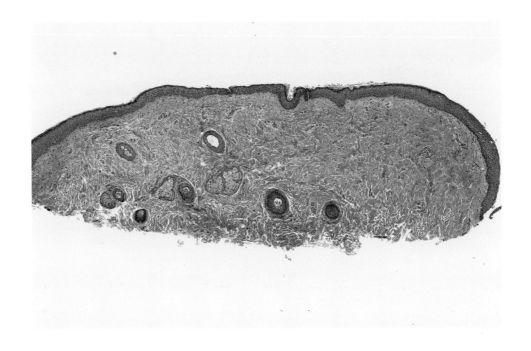

Diagnosis: Limbal dermoid.

Clinical description: Slit-lamp examination reveals an elevated yellow mass with associated cilia straddling the temporal limbus.

Histological description: Histopathology reveals tissue lined by keratinized stratified squamous epithelium with associated pilosebaceous units. The underlying dermis is fibrotic.

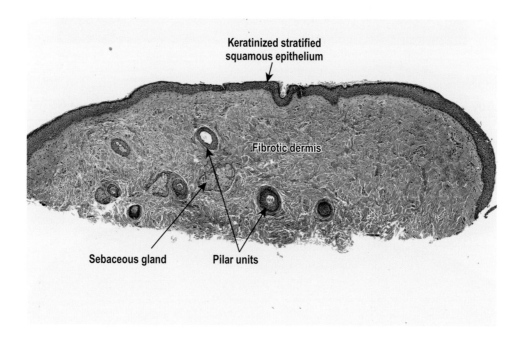

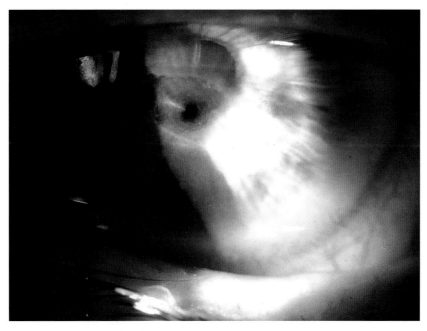

Courtesy of Neal P. Barney, M.D. University of Wisconsin-Madison.

A 63-year-old woman with a history of rheumatoid arteritis presented with central corneal thinning.

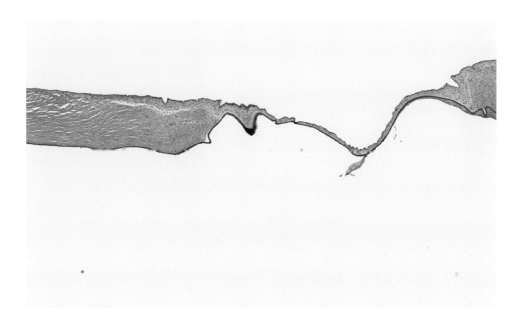

Diagnosis: Descemetocele.

Clinical description: Slit-lamp examination shows a central area of corneal thinning consistent with Descemetocele.

Histological description: Histopathology shows complete loss of the stroma centrally. Only Descemet's membrane and an attenuated epithelium remain in this area.

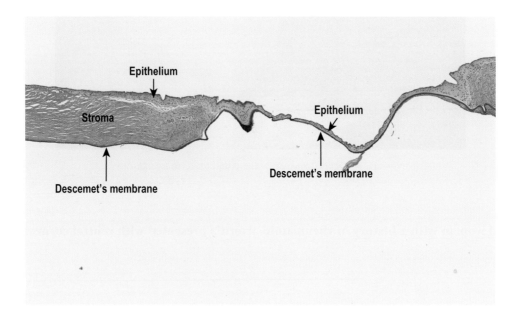

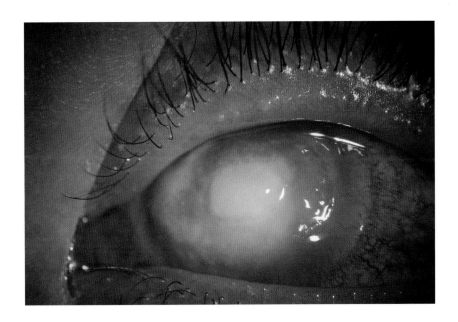

A 32-year-old contact lens wearer presented with a longstanding central corneal ulcer. The ulcer was treated with fortified antibiotic eye drops with no response. Corneal cultures were negative for bacteria, fungus, and acanthamoeba. Therapeutic penetrating keratoplasty was performed.

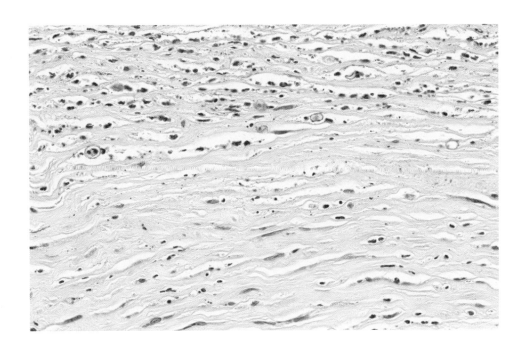

Diagnosis: Acanthamoeba keratitis.

Clinical description: Central corneal infiltrate is seen. There are multiple satellite lesions surrounding the main infiltrate. The remaining cornea is edematous.

Histological description: The corneal tissue is infiltrated with round, double wall cysts of acanthamoeba (arrows). Infiltration with neutrophils is also seen.

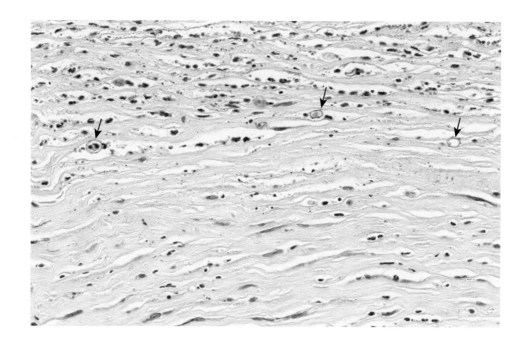

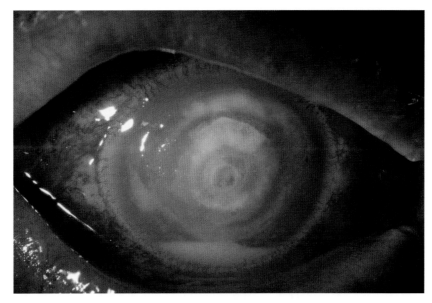

Courtesy of Sarah M. Nehls, M.D. University of Wisconsin-Madison.

A 63-year-old farmer presented with a corneal ulcer and hypopyon. The condition worsened despite topical antifungal therapy. He subsequently underwent a penetrating keratoplasty.

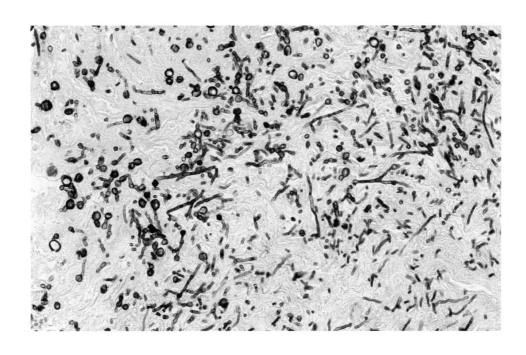

Diagnosis: Fungal keratitis secondary to *Aspergillus*.

Clinical description: Slit-lamp examination reveals a central corneal infiltrate with feathery edges. A 3-mm hypopyon is present.

Histological description: Gomori methenamine silver (GMS) stain demonstrates septated branching filamentous fungi. The branching is at 45-degree angles (circles) consistent with *Aspergillus*.

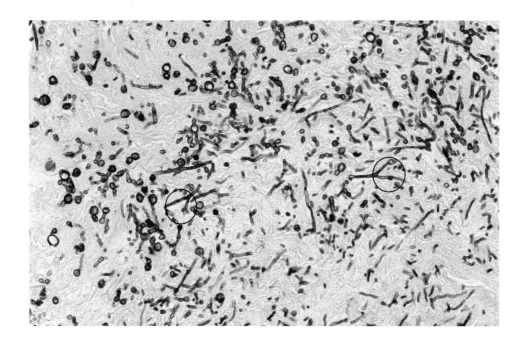

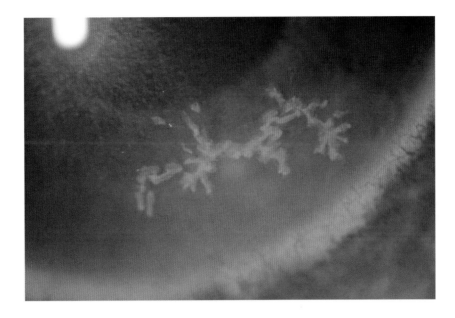

A 36-year-old man presented with ocular pain and photophobia. The slit-lamp examination is seen above. Later he developed corneal scarring and decreased vision.

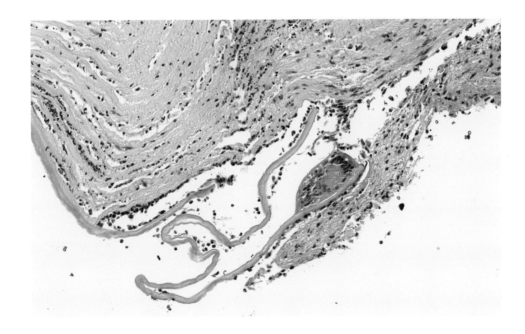

Diagnosis: Herpes simplex virus (HSV) keratitis.

Clinical description: Corneal dendritic lesions with terminal bulbs are seen.

Histological description: A marked inflammatory response in the posterior cornea is present. The Descemet's membrane is fragmented. Epithelioid and multinucleated giant cells are also present in the area of Descemet's membrane.

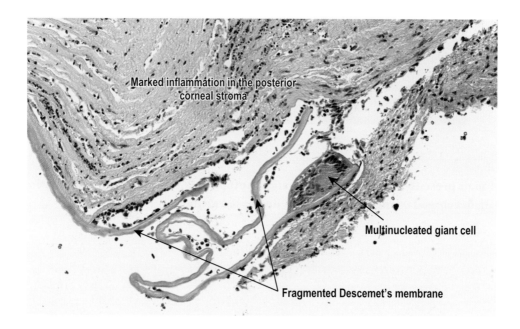

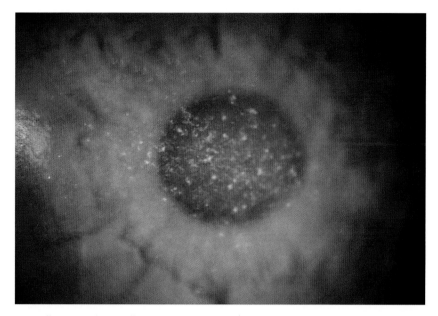

From Albert, Daniel M., Miller, Joan W., Azar, Dimitri T., and Blodi, Barbara A. (eds). 2008. Albert
& Jakobiec's Principles and Practice of Ophthalmology, 3rd ed. Philadelphia: Copyright Elsevier 2008.

A 42-year-old man with AIDS presented with decreased vision and corneal changes.

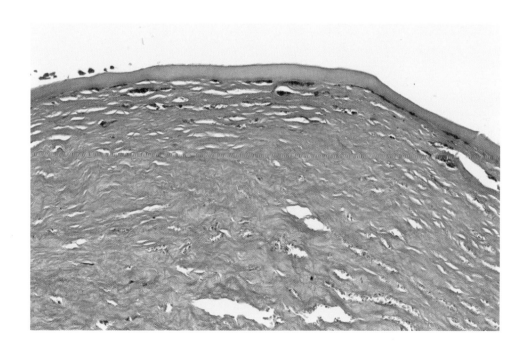

Diagnosis: Microsporidial keratitis.

Clinical description: Slit-lamp examination demonstrates multiple punctate corneal opacities.

Histological description: Histopathological evaluation of the corneal tissue demonstrates anterior stromal deposits consistent with microsporidia (arrows).

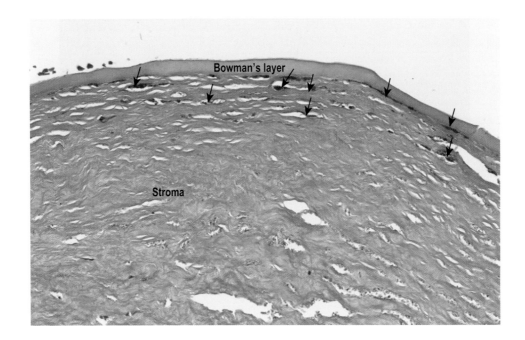

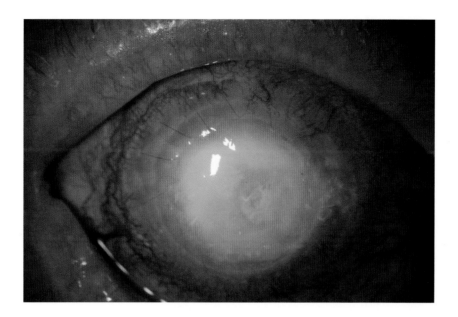

A 53-year-old man with a history of corneal transplant presented with a corneal infiltrate not responding to topical antibiotics. He had several previous penetrating keratoplasties.

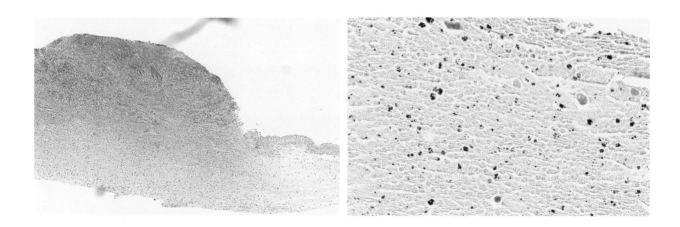

Diagnosis: Bacterial keratitis due to MRSA (methicillin resistant *Staphylococcus aureus*).

Clinical description: Slit-lamp examination demonstrates a central corneal infiltrate with an overlying epithelial defect.

Histological description: Corneal tissue is infiltrated with numerous neutrophils (top). Gram stain demonstrates scattered clusters of Gram-positive cocci (arrows).

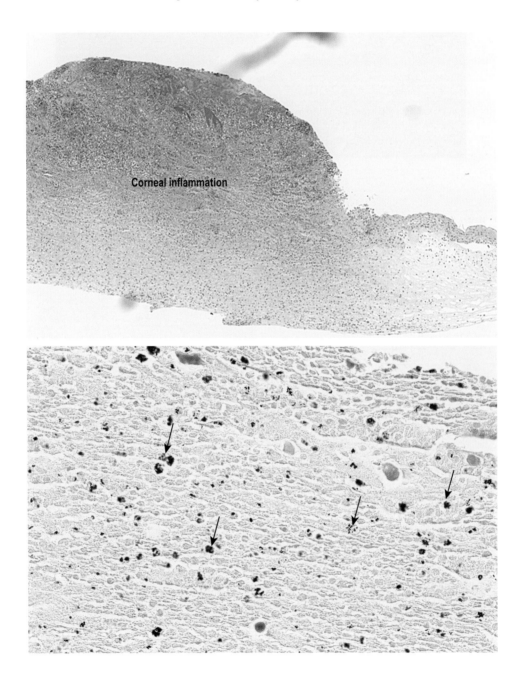

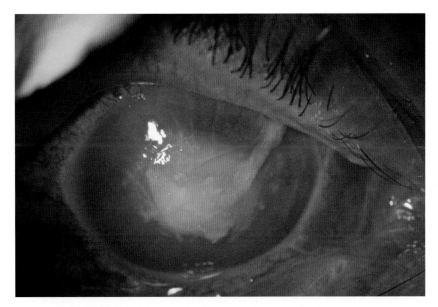

Printed with permission from Azari A.A., Nehls S., Ghoghawala S.Y., Lee V., Kanavi M.R., Potter H.D. Rhizopus Keratitis Following Corneal Trauma. JAMA Ophthalmology 2013; 131(6):776.

A 48-year-old man presented with a central corneal ulcer after trauma with a metal wire.

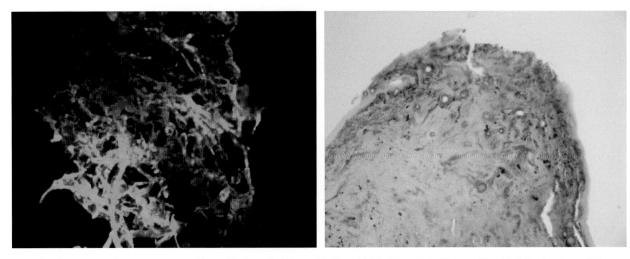

Printed with permission from Azari A.A., Nehls S., Ghoghawala S.Y., Lee V., Kanavi M.R., Potter H.D. Rhizopus Keratitis Following Corneal Trauma. JAMA Ophthalmology 2013; 131(6):776.

Diagnosis: Rhizopus keratitis.

Clinical description: Slit-lamp examination shows a central necrotic corneal ulcer with an overlying epithelial defect.

Histological description: Branching filamentous fungi are seen demonstrating an exquisite pattern of autofluorescence (top). Microscopic evaluation demonstrates multiple branching nonseptate hyphae (arrows, bottom).

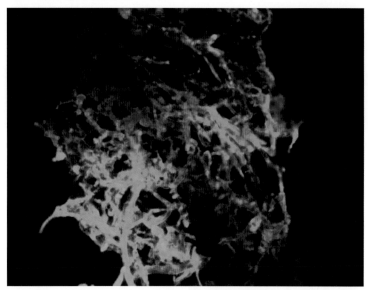

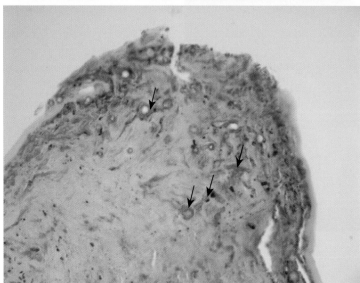

Printed with permission from Azari A.A., Nehls S., Ghoghawala S.Y., Lee V., Kanavi M.R., Potter H.D. Rhizopus Keratitis Following Corneal Trauma. JAMA Ophthalmology 2013; 131(6):776.

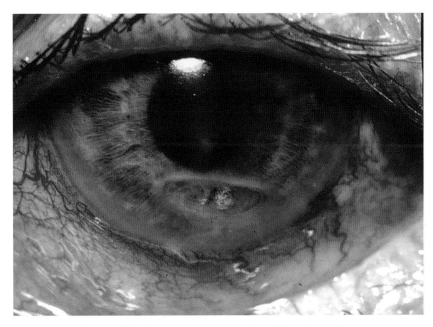

Courtesy of Neal P. Barney, M.D. University of Wisconsin-Madison.

A 43-year-old woman with past history of ocular shingles presented with a nonhealing corneal ulcer.

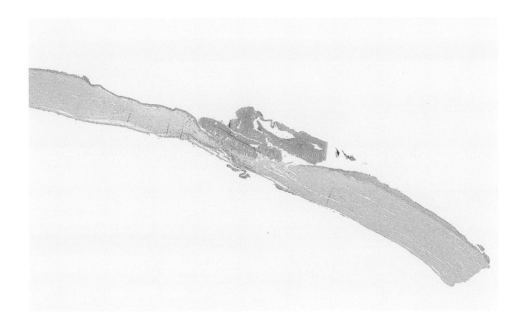

Diagnosis: Herpes zoster keratitis.

Clinical description: Nonhealing corneal ulcer.

Histological description: Histopathology reveals central corneal thinning (double headed arrow) with marked inflammation. An overlying epithelial defect, consistent with neurotrophic ulcer, is present.

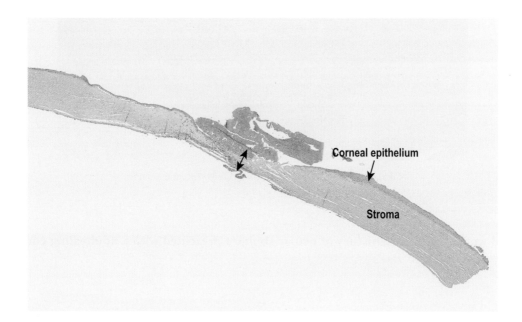

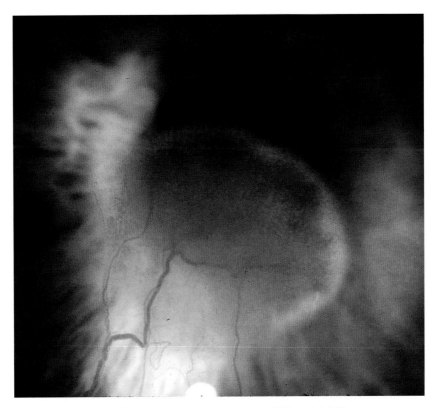

Courtesy of Neal P. Barney, M.D. University of Wisconsin-Madison.

A 45-year-old woman presented with decreased vision and corneal neovascularization as shown above.

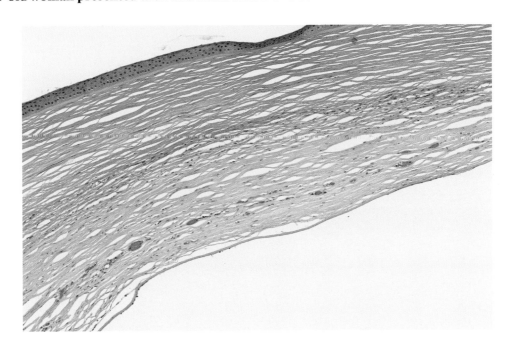

Diagnosis: Interstitial keratitis.

Clinical description: Slit-lamp examination demonstrates a round area of corneal opacity with neovascularization.

Histological description: Marked inflammation, vascularization, and scarring are seen in the posterior third of the cornea.

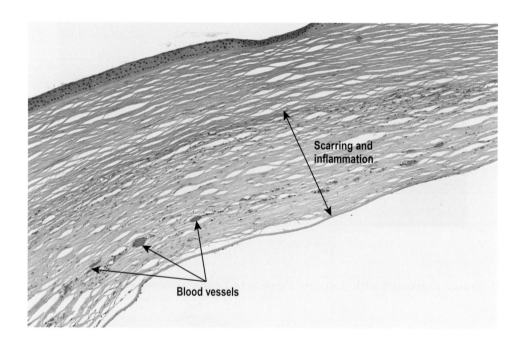

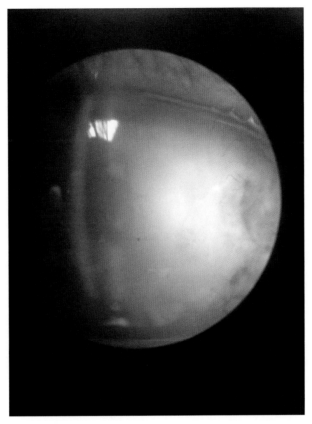

Courtesy of Matthew J. Thompson, Tower Clock Eye Center, Green Bay, WI.

A 77-year-old man presented with corneal neovascularization and opacity unresponsive to topical and subconjunctival steroids. He subsequently underwent an enucleation.

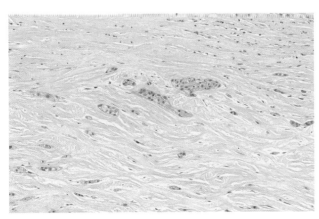

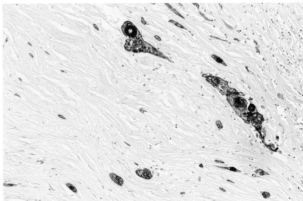

Diagnosis: Corneal squamous cell carcinoma.

Clinical description: Examination with the slit-lamp demonstrates corneal scar and whitening.

Histological description: Histopathology shows an edematous cornea infiltrated with epithelioid cells with severe atypia (arrows, top) staining with cytokeratin AE1/AE3, a marker for squamous cells (arrows, bottom).

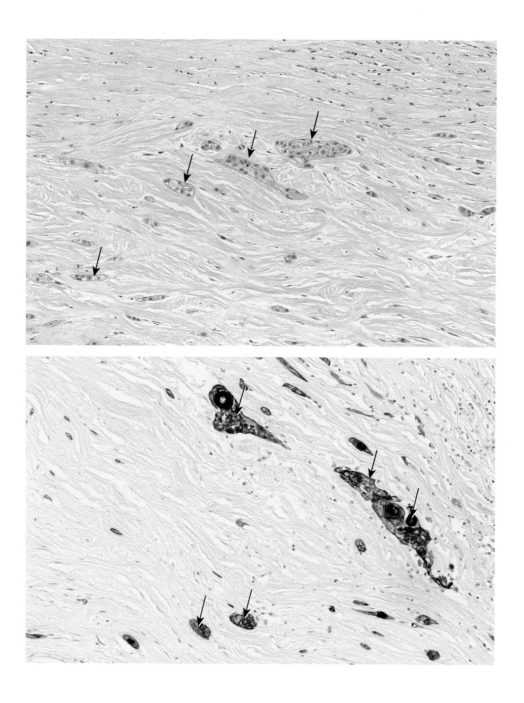

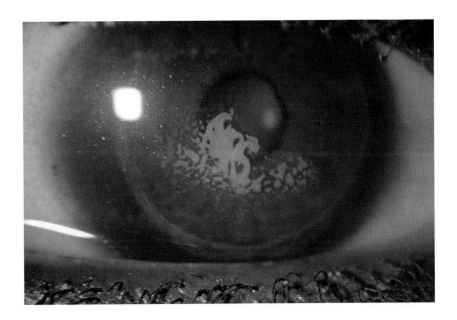

A 65-year-old man presented with the above corneal changes 6 months after a complicated cataract surgery.

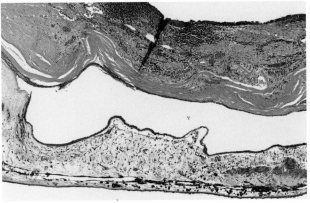
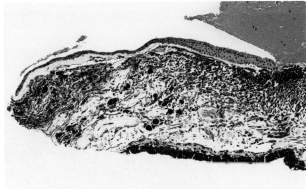

Diagnosis: Epithelial ingrowth.

Clinical description: Epithelial ingrowth causing corneal haze is evident. The leading edge of the epithelial ingrowth has scalloped borders.

Histological description: Growth of nonkeratinized stratified squamous epithelium on the posterior surface of the cornea as well as anterior iris is shown.

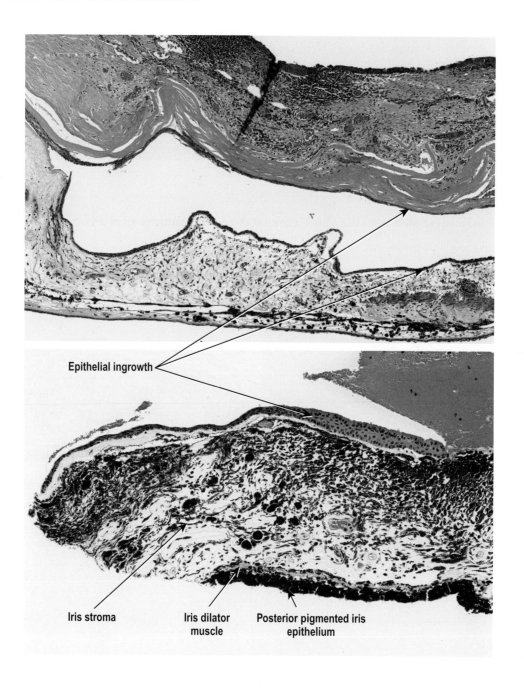

Epithelial ingrowth

Iris stroma   Iris dilator muscle   Posterior pigmented iris epithelium

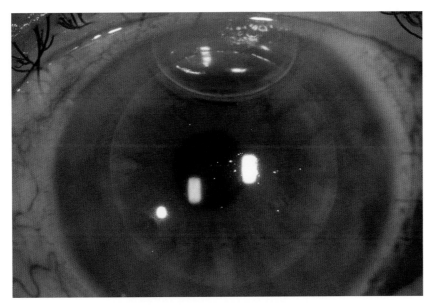

From Albert, Daniel M., Miller, Joan W., Azar, Dimitri T., and Blodi, Barbara A. (eds). 2008. Albert & Jakobiec's Principles and Practice of Ophthalmology, 3rd ed. Philadelphia: Copyright Elsevier 2008.

A 68-year-old man with a history of Fuchs' endothelial dystrophy was seen in the clinic on postoperative day 1, after a Descemet's stripping endothelial keratoplasty (DSEK).

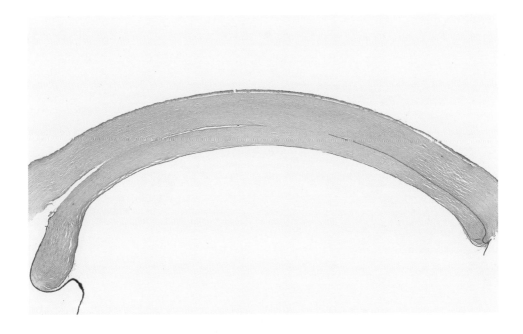

Diagnosis: Corneal button demonstrating a failed DSEK procedure obtained after full thickness corneal transplant.

Clinical description: Slit-lamp examination reveals an eye after DSEK surgery with graft in a good central position. A small air bubble remains superiorly, but usually resolves in 2–3 days.

Histological description: Histopathology demonstrates a traditional full thickness corneal transplant performed after failed DSEK surgery. Host Descemet's membrane is present at the donor–recipient interface.

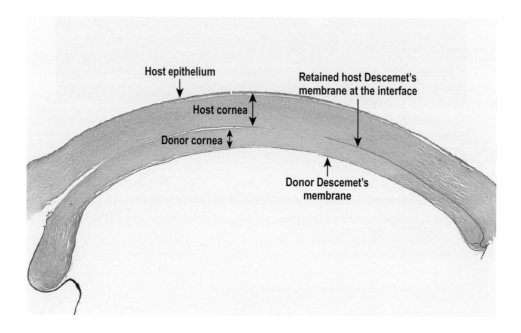

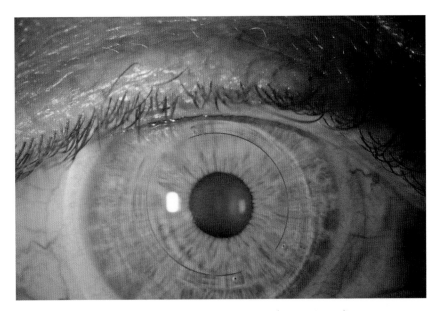

Courtesy of Sarah M. Nehls, M.D. University of Wisconsin-Madison.

A 43-year-old man with progressive keratoconus presented with the above clinical picture 1 month postoperatively. Many years later, he required a corneal transplant.

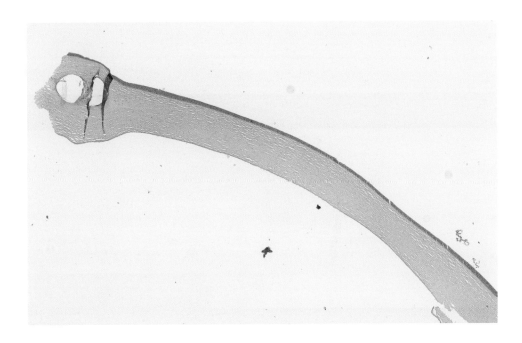

Diagnosis: Intrastromal corneal ring segments (INTACS) in an eye with a history of keratoconus.

Clinical description: Slit-lamp examination demonstrates two INTACS placed superiorly and inferiorly.

Histological description: Histopathology demonstrates a thinned cornea with an intrastromal defect where the INTACS were placed (asterisk).

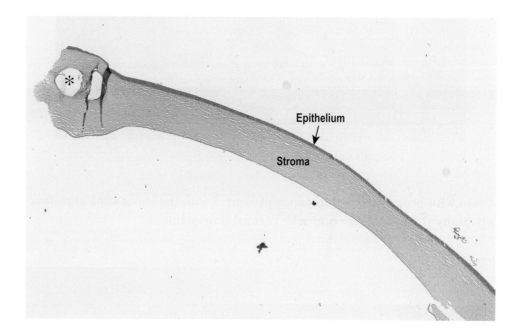

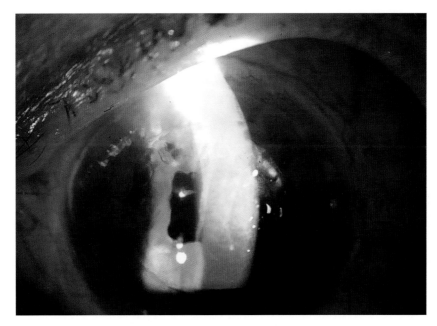

Courtesy of Neal P. Barney, M.D. University of Wisconsin-Madison.

A 48-year-old male patient has a longstanding history of corneal edema and decreased vision no longer amenable to medical therapy. He underwent penetrating keratoplasty.

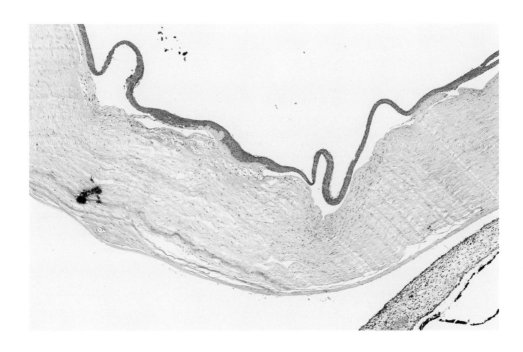

Diagnosis: Pseudophakic bullous keratopathy.

Clinical description: Slit-lamp examination demonstrates marked corneal haze and edema.

Histological description: The cornea is thickened. Areas of separation between the epithelium and the Bowman's layer are seen (asterisk).

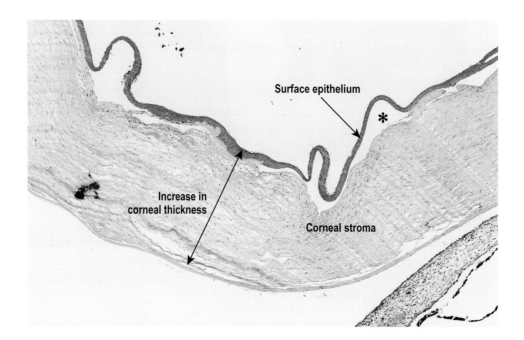

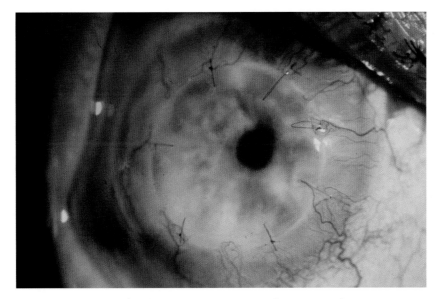

Courtesy of Neal P. Barney, M.D. University of Wisconsin-Madison.

A 48-year-old man presented with decreased vision and photophobia 2 years following a corneal transplant.

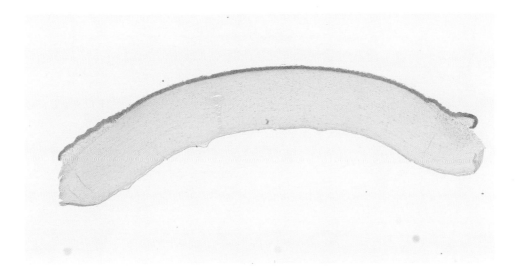

Diagnosis: Failed corneal graft.

Clinical description: A hazy and edematous cornea with areas of neovascularization is seen.

Histological description: The corneal tissue is edematous with loss of natural stromal clefts. Areas of inflammation, particularly at the edges of the transplant, are apparent.

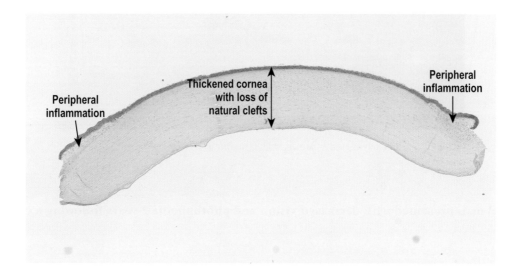

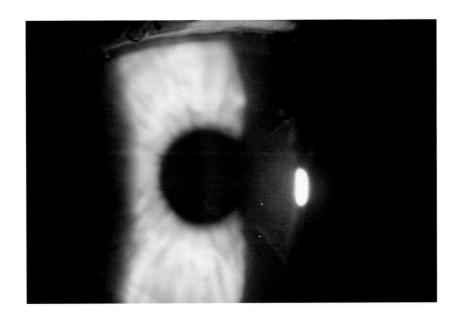

A 48-year-old man presented with irregular astigmatism uncorrected with rigid gas permeable lenses. He underwent penetrating keratoplasty.

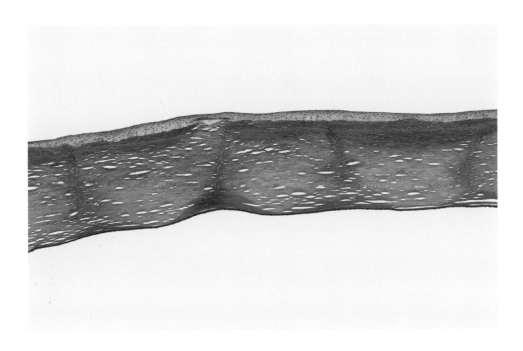

Diagnosis: Previous radial keratotomy.

Clinical description: Multiple radially oriented linear corneal scars consistent with radial keratotomy are seen.

Histological description: Histopathology demonstrates multiple partial thickness corneal scars (arrowheads).

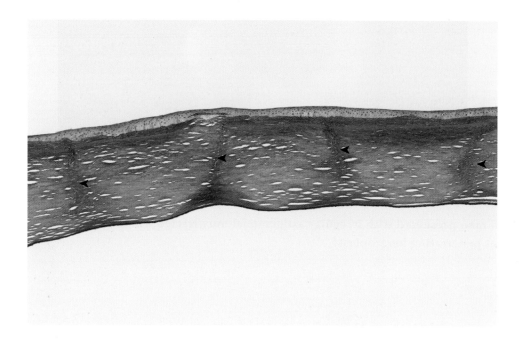

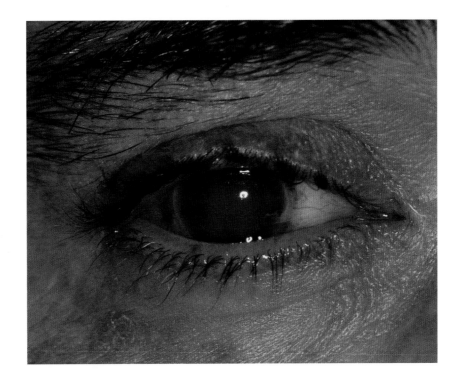

A 54-year-old male presented with corneal clouding 2 months after injury with a softball. The corneal clouding did not resolve and he underwent a penetrating keratoplasty.

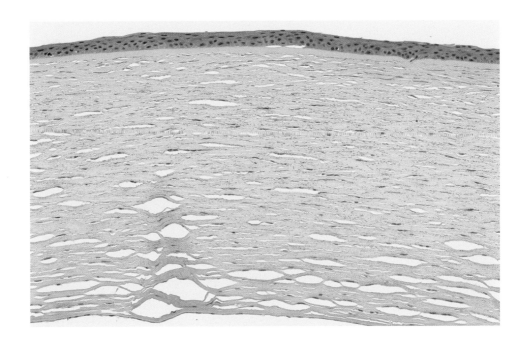

Diagnosis: Corneal blood staining.

Clinical description: Corneal blood staining and opacification are seen.

Histological description: Red blood cells are seen scattered within an edematous cornea.

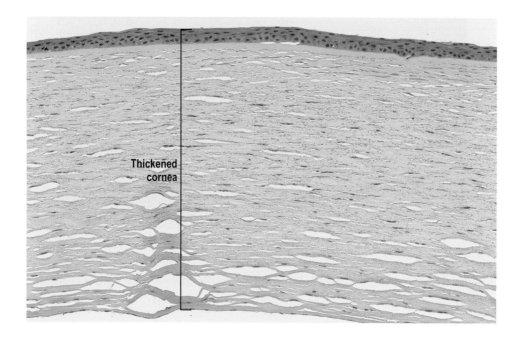

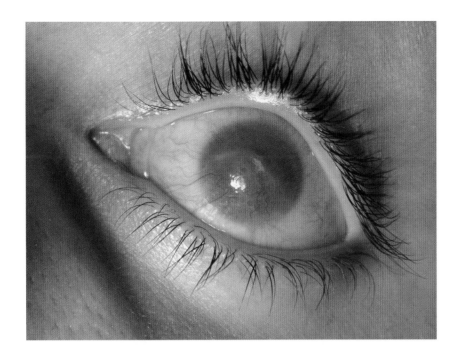

The patient is a 20-year-old man with history of chemical burn of the left eye from propionic acid. He underwent stem cell transplant. The specimen below was removed from his corneal surface.

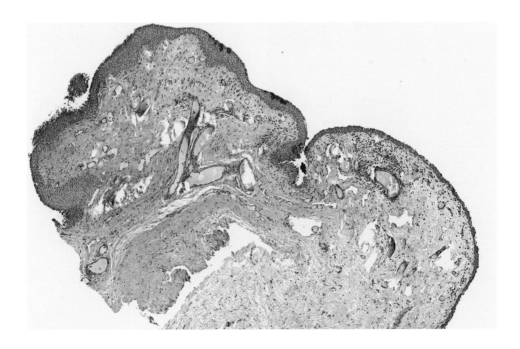

Diagnosis: Corneal conjunctivalization secondary to stem cell deficiency.

Clinical description: Clinical examination reveals corneal haze and pannus secondary to stem cell deficiency.

Histological description: Histopathology reveals goblet cells containing nonkeratinized stratified squamous epithelium of the conjunctiva overlying a loose, highly vascularized (asterisks) substantia propria with lymphoplasmacytic infiltrate (arrowheads).

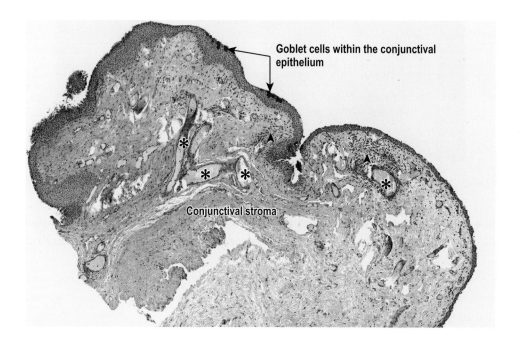

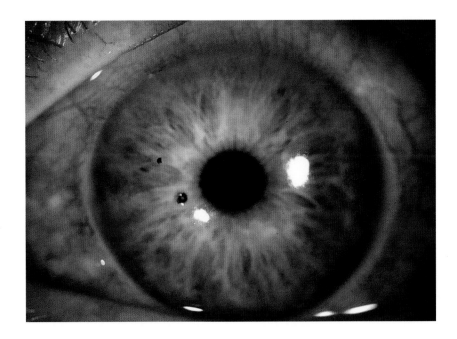

A 38-year-old man presented with tearing, redness, and pain in his left eye after working in his garage.

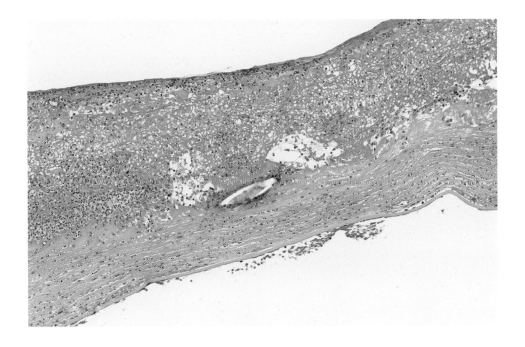

Diagnosis: Corneal foreign body.

Clinical description: A foreign body with a surrounding rust ring is seen embedded within the cornea.

Histological description: The cornea demonstrates profound scarring and inflammation. There is loss of keratocytes and stromal disorganization within the anterior two-thirds of the cornea. Foreign body material is noted.

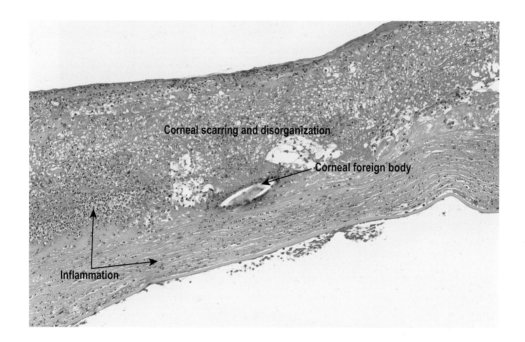

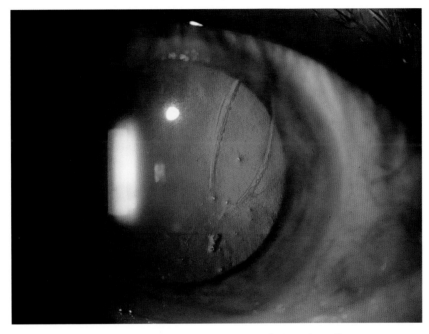

Courtesy of Neal P. Barney, M.D. University of Wisconsin-Madison.

A 12-year-old boy with a history of forceps delivery presented with the above corneal finding. He underwent a penetrating keratoplasty many years later.

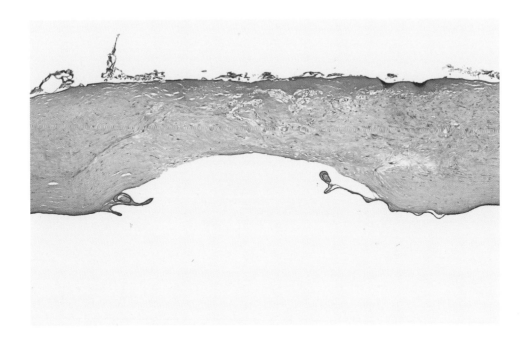

Diagnosis: Vertical breaks in the Descemet's membrane in a patient with a history of forceps delivery.

Clinical description: Vertical breaks in the Descemet's membrane are noted.

Histological description: Histopathology reveals a scarred corneal stroma. The surface epithelium is largely missing. There is a break in the Descemet's membrane with scrolling of this membrane.

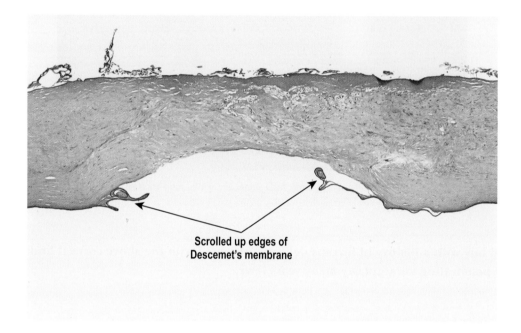

Scrolled up edges of
Descemet's membrane

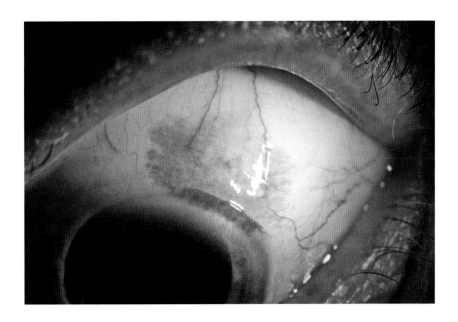

A 42-year-old woman presented with a new conjunctival lesion as shown above. She underwent excisional biopsy of her conjunctival lesion.

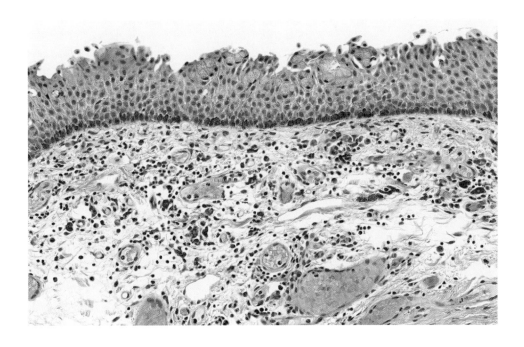

Diagnosis: Primary acquired melanosis (PAM) without atypia.

Clinical description: A flat pigmented lesion on the superior bulbar conjunctiva is seen.

Histological description: Histopathology reveals conjunctiva with mild acanthosis. There is an increased number of bland-appearing pigmented melanocytes along the basal epithelial layer (arrowheads). There is no atypia, no melanocytic nesting nor intraepithelial spread.

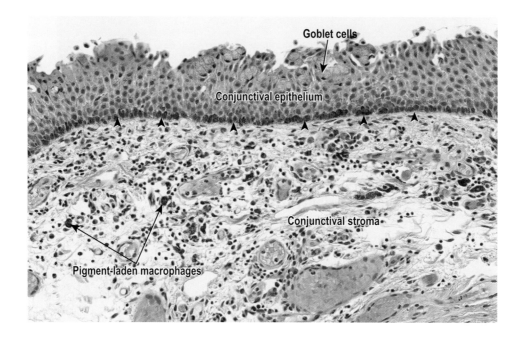

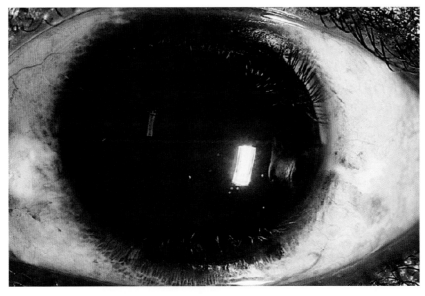

From Albert, Daniel M., Miller, Joan W., Azar, Dimitri T., and Blodi, Barbara A. (eds) 2008. Albert
& Jakobiec's Principles and Practice of Ophthalmology, 3rd ed. Philadelphia: Copyright Elsevier 2008.

**A 49-year-old woman presented with darkly pigmented conjunctival lesions as shown above. She later
underwent conjunctival biopsy.**

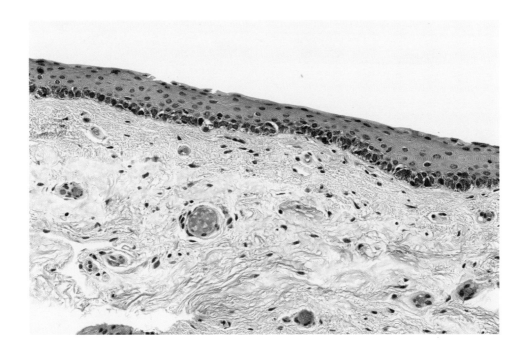

Diagnosis: Benign acquired melanosis (BAM), also known as racial melanosis.

Clinical description: The clinical examination reveals multiple pigmented conjunctival lesions.

Histological description: Histopathology demonstrates tissue lined by nonkeratinized stratified squamous epithelium with an increased number of bland-appearing pigmented melanocytes along the basal epithelial layer (arrows).

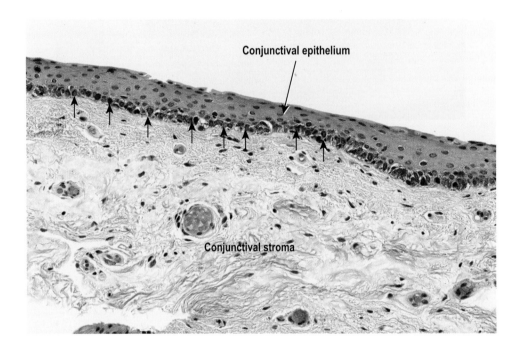

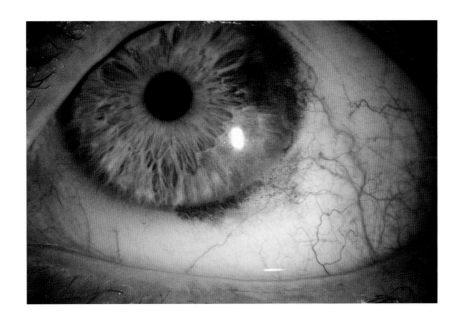

A 48-year-old Caucasian woman presented with the pigmented lesions as shown above.

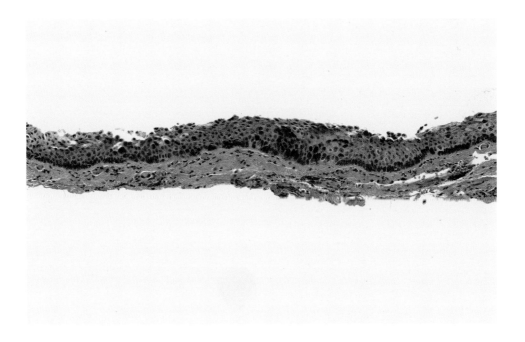

Diagnosis: Primary acquired melanosis (PAM) with atypia.

Clinical description: Conjunctival pigmentation is seen in the lateral limbus spanning an area approximating four clock hours.

Histological description: Histopathological evaluation demonstrates involvement of the superficial (arrows), as well as deep (arrowheads) epithelium, with pigmented melanocytes.

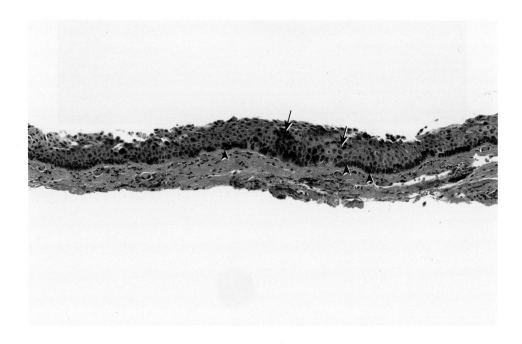

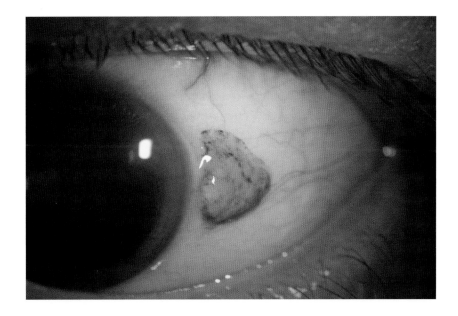

A 14-year-old girl presented with a slow-growing conjunctival lesion. The lesion has continued to enlarge in recent years.

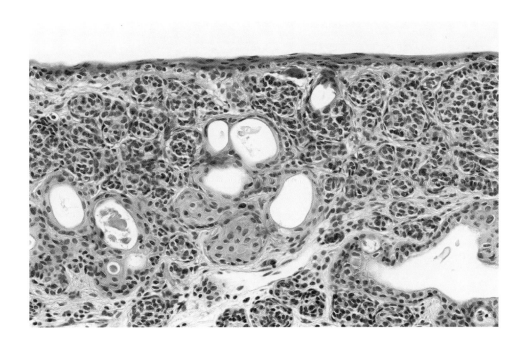

Diagnosis: Conjunctival nevus.

Clinical description: A raised, cystic, pigmented bulbar conjunctival lesion is seen on clinical examination.

Histological description: Histopathology reveals a nonkeratinized stratified squamous epithelium. Nests of melanocytes (arrowheads) are seen below the epithelium. Multiple epithelial-lined cysts are also present (asterisks).

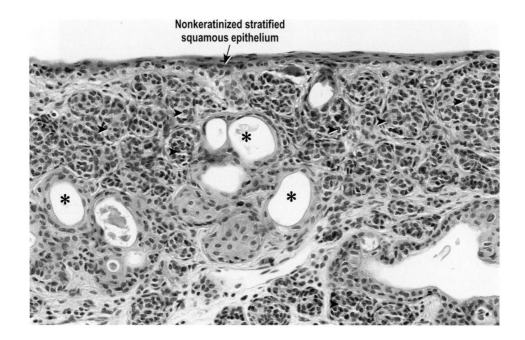

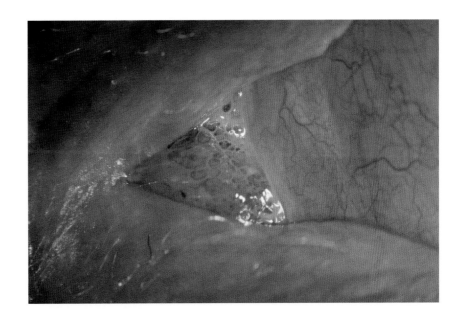

An 84-year-old man presented with a 2-year history of a left caruncular lesion. He underwent excisional biopsy of the lesion.

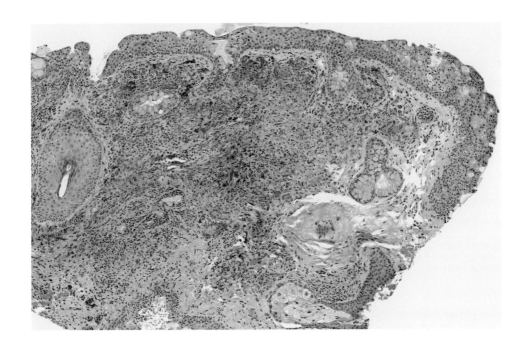

Diagnosis: Caruncular nevus.

Clinical description: Slit-lamp examination reveals a pigmented caruncular lesion.

Histological description: The slides reveal nonkeratinized stratified squamous epithelium with goblet cells and associated pilosebaceous units. Nests of melanocytic cells with variable pigmentation are seen within the stroma.

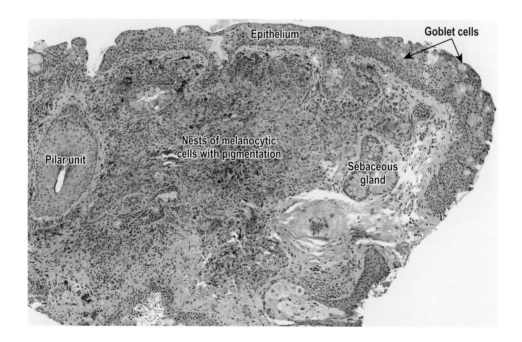

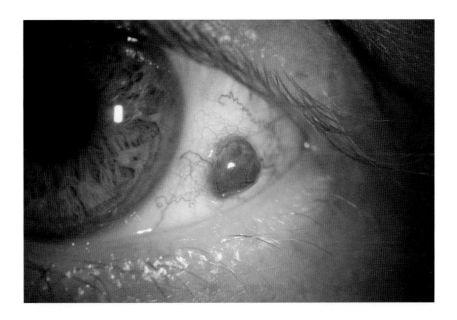

A 66-year-old man presented with a darkly pigmented conjunctival lesion. An excisional biopsy was performed.

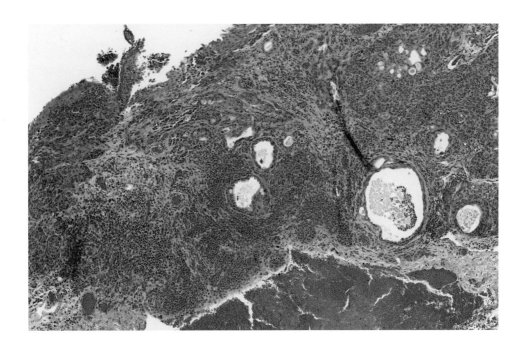

Diagnosis: Conjunctival melanoma arising from nevus.

Clinical description: Anterior segment examination reveals a raised, darkly pigmented conjunctival lesion with feeder vessels.

Histological description: The conjunctival epithelium (asterisk) and stroma is infiltrated with melanocytic cells (arrows) with associated epithelial inclusion cysts. Some of these melanocytic cells are arranged in nests, while others demonstrate marked pleomorphism and prominent nucleoli.

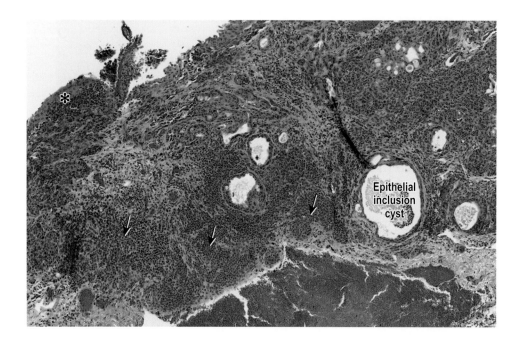

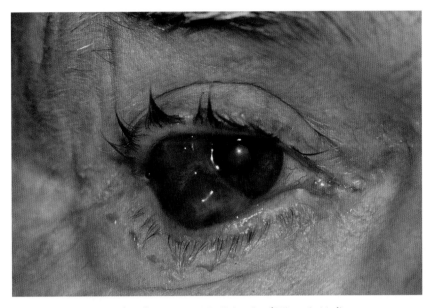

Courtesy of Neal P. Barney, M.D. University of Wisconsin-Madison.

An 87-year-old woman presented with the above clinical picture. Two years earlier the patient was diagnosed with a skin melanoma in her thumb.

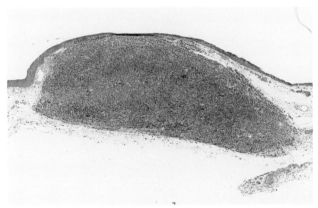

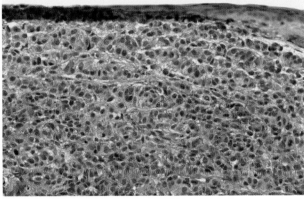

Diagnosis: Metastatic conjunctival melanoma.

Clinical description: Slit-lamp examination demonstrates a large raised conjunctival mass.

Histological description: The conjunctival tissue is infiltrated with clusters of large atypical melanocytes with prominent nucleoli and pigmentation.

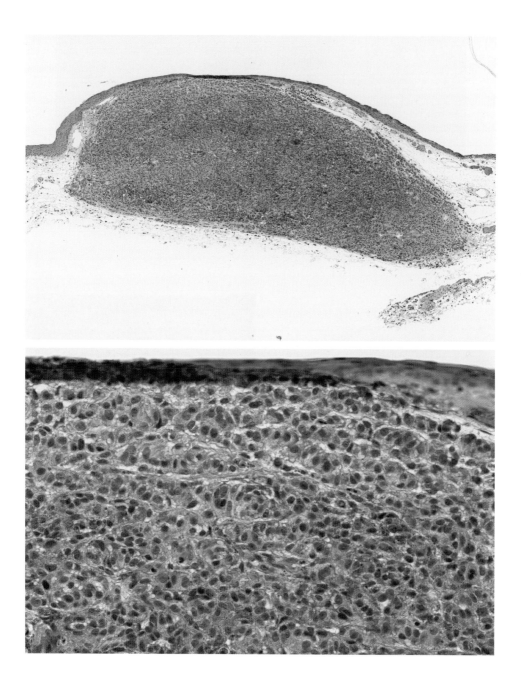

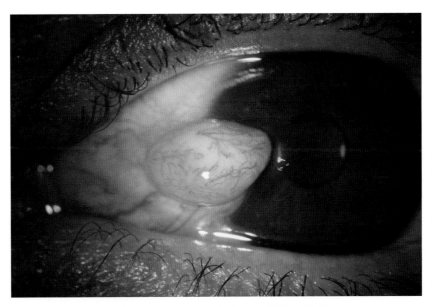

Courtesy of Neal P. Barney, M.D. University of Wisconsin-Madison.

A 23-year-old man presented with a 2-year history of a slow growing left eye lesion. He underwent excisional biopsy of the eyelid lesion.

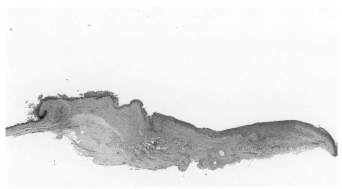

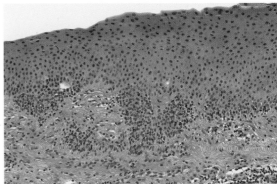

Diagnosis: Pterygium and nevus occurring in the same area.

Clinical description: Clinical examination reveals a vascularized, balloon-like mass straddling the limbus, nasally.

Histological description: Histopathological examination demonstrates conjunctival epithelium with solar elastosis, consistent with a pterygium (left side, asterisk), and proliferation of melanocytic cells in the stroma and epithelial–stromal interface, consistent with a junctional nevus (right side, arrows).

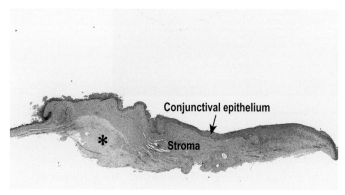
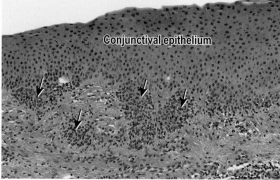

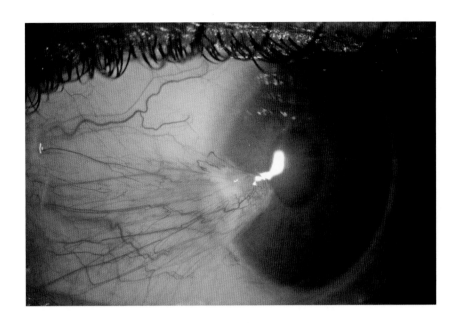

A 44-year-old Hispanic man presented with a growing lesion in his left eye.

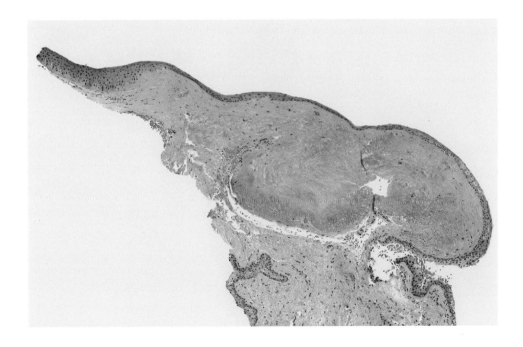

Diagnosis: Pterygium.

Clinical description: The clinical examination reveals a vascular "insect wing-like" growth over the nasal cornea.

Histological description: Histopathology reveals a lesion with nonkeratinized stratified epithelium. Solar elastotic changes are present within the stroma (asterisks). A fragment of the cornea is also present.

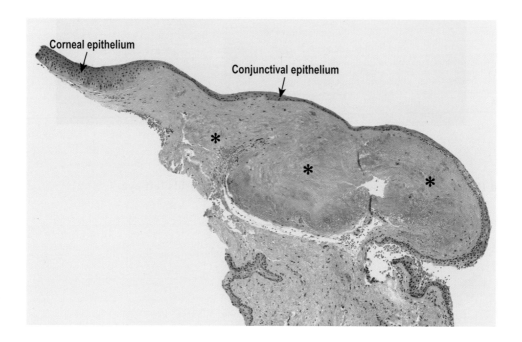

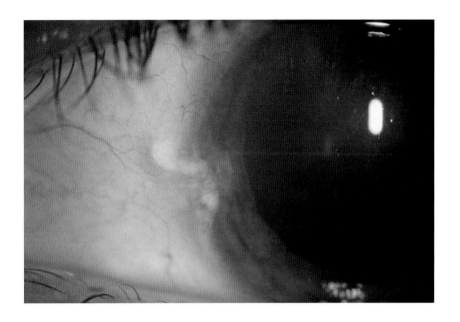

A 32-year-old man presented with a raised conjunctival lesion.

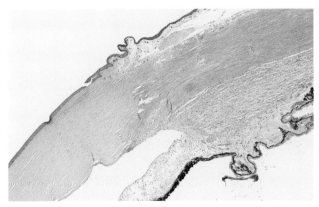 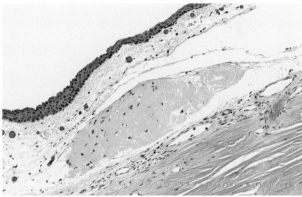

Diagnosis: Pinguecula.

Clinical description: Clinical examination reveals an elevated lesion with mild leukoplakia.

Histological description: Histopathology demonstrates solar elastotic changes (asterisk) within the conjunctival stroma.

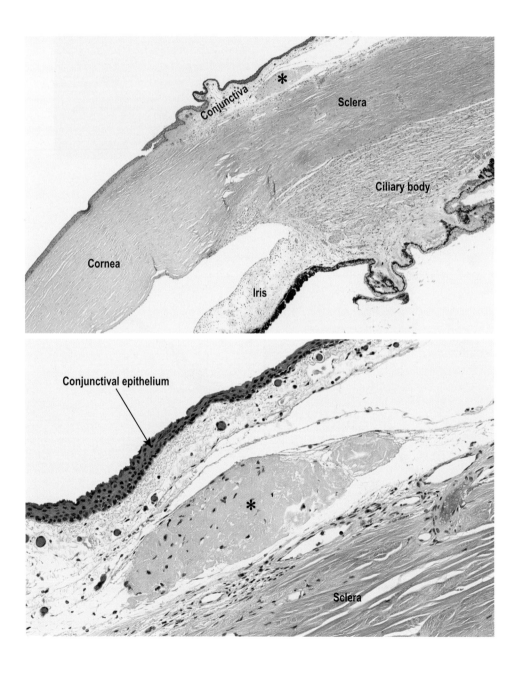

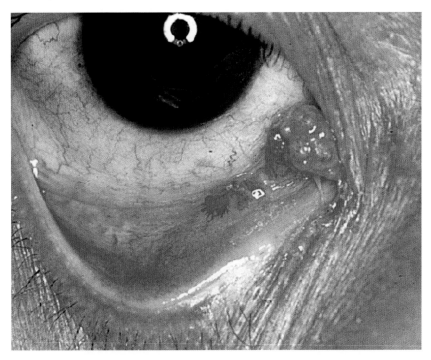

From Albert, Daniel M., Miller, Joan W., Azar, Dimitri T., and Blodi, Barbara A. (eds). 2008. Albert & Jakobiec's Principles and Practice of Ophthalmology, 3rd ed. Philadelphia: Copyright Elsevier 2008.

A 79-year-old woman presented with ocular discomfort and epiphora.

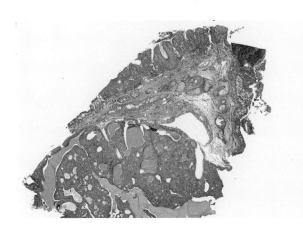

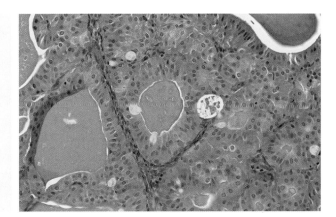

Diagnosis: Oncocytoma.

Clinical description: Slit-lamp examination shows an elevated round caruncular lesion.

Histological description: Low power histopathology (top) reveals tissue lined by goblet-cell-containing nonkeratinized, stratified squamous epithelium with associated pilosebaceous units. Underlying the surface epithelium, sheets of epithelial cells forming ductal and glandular structures (arrowheads) that contain PAS positive material within their lumen are seen (asterisks, bottom). The epithelial cells exhibit a granular eosinophilic cytoplasm.

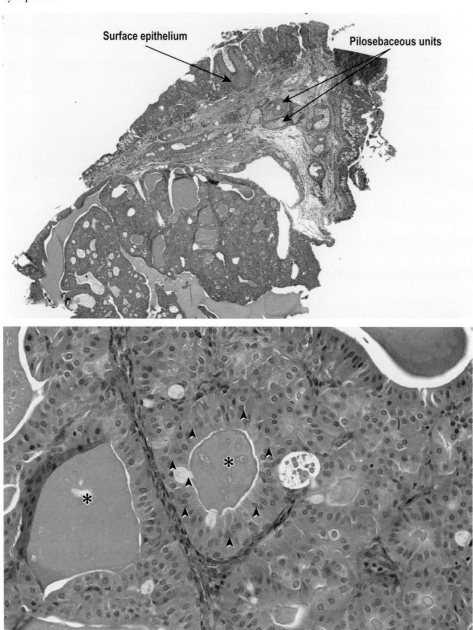

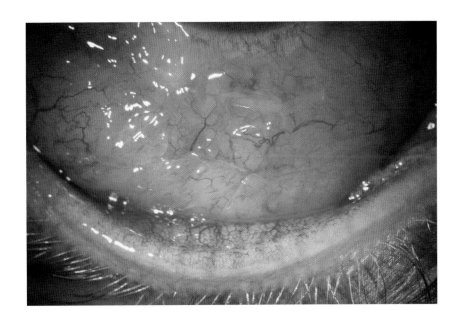

A 31-year-old man presented with increased redness and discomfort in his right eye. A biopsy was performed. The hematoxylin and eosin stain is on the left; the Congo red stain is on the right.

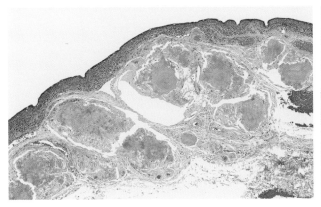 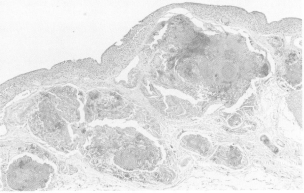

Diagnosis: Conjunctival amyloidosis.

Clinical description: The slit-lamp examination demonstrates a yellow elevated lesion on the inferior bulbar conjunctiva.

Histological description: The slides reveal a specimen covered by conjunctival epithelium. There are numerous, large amorphous eosinophilic deposits in the stroma (top). The eosinophilic material stains with Congo red (bottom) and displays dichroism under polarized light (not shown).

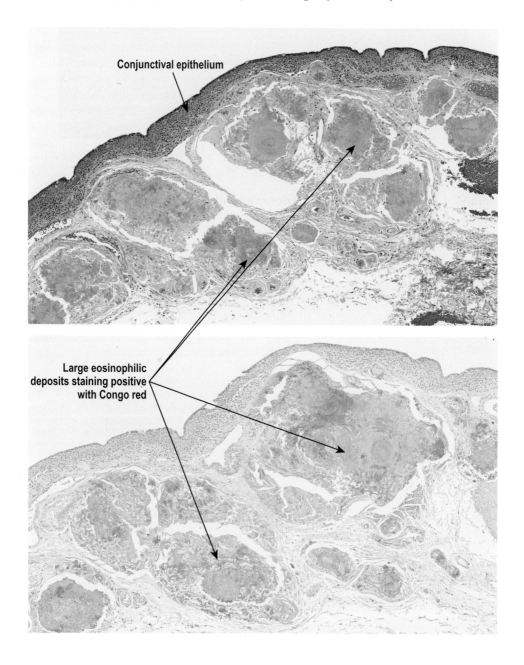

Conjunctival epithelium

Large eosinophilic deposits staining positive with Congo red

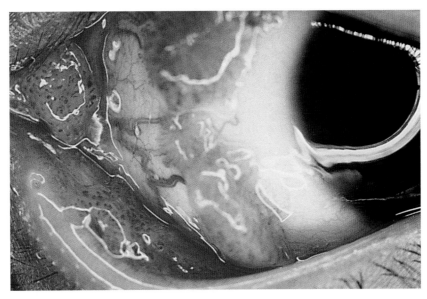

From Albert, Daniel M., Miller, Joan W., Azar, Dimitri T., and Blodi, Barbara A. (eds). 2008. Albert & Jakobiec's Principles and Practice of Ophthalmology, 3rd ed. Philadelphia: Copyright Elsevier 2008.

A 7-year-old boy presented with left eye discomfort and excessive tearing.

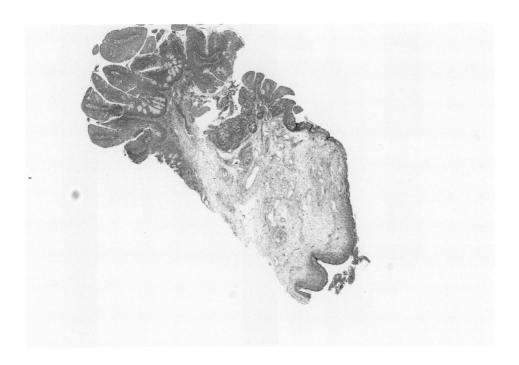

Diagnosis: Conjunctival squamous papilloma.

Clinical description: Slit-lamp examination demonstrates several papillomatous conjunctival lesions located nasally.

Histological description: Histopathology reveals tissue lined by nonkeratinized stratified squamous epithelium containing goblet cells. There are multiple papillary fronds (circles) of acanthotic nonkeratinized stratified squamous epithelium.

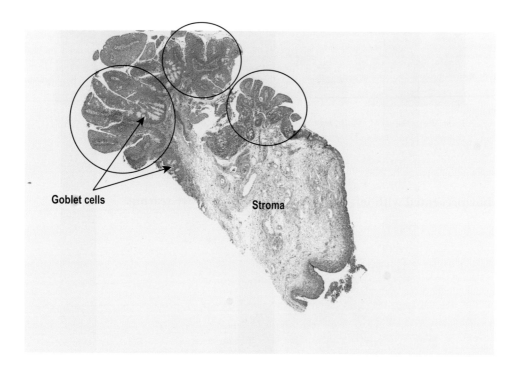

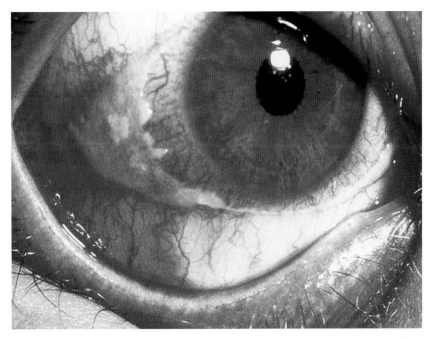

From Albert, Daniel M., Miller, Joan W., Azar, Dimitri T., and Blodi, Barbara A. (eds). 2008. Albert & Jakobiec's Principles and Practice of Ophthalmology, 3rd ed. Philadelphia: Copyright Elsevier 2008.

A 26-year-old Native American man presented with a conjunctival lesion.

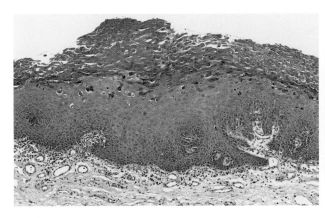
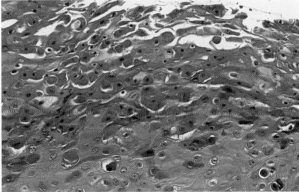

Diagnosis: Hereditary benign intraepithelial dyskeratosis (HBID).

Clinical description: A clinical photograph demonstrates a limbal leukoplakic lesion in this patient.

Histological description: Histopathology demonstrates hyperkeratosis, acanthosis, parakeratosis, and dyskeratosis (keratin within the individual epithelial cells, shown with asterisks in the bottom image).

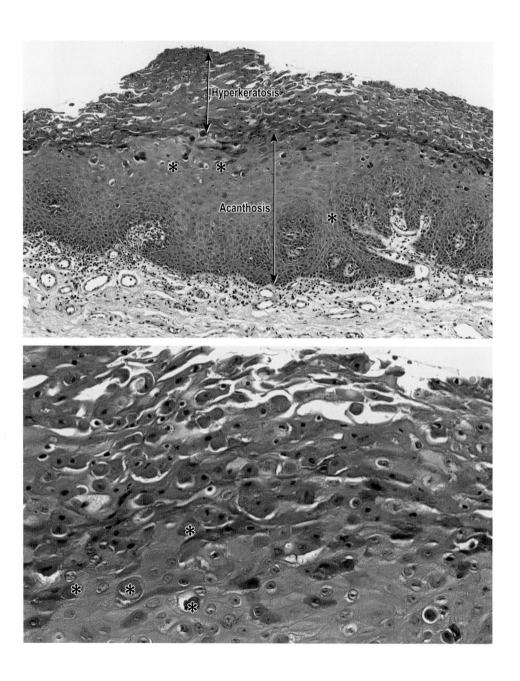

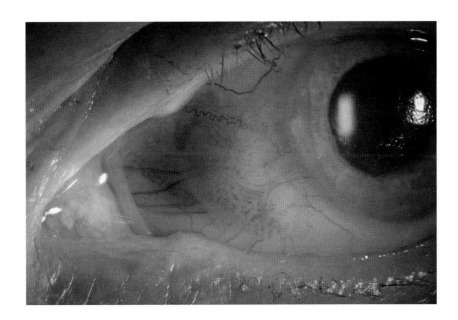

A 44-year-old man presented with a newly-formed lesion in his left eye. The lesion appeared approximately 3 months ago and it has been increasing in size.

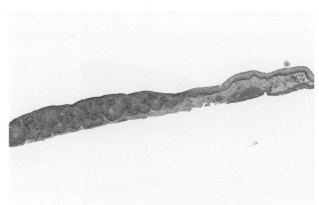

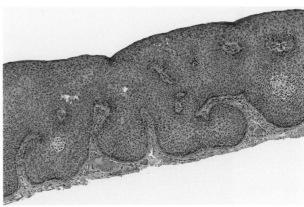

Diagnosis: Conjunctival intraepithelial neoplasia (CIN).

Clinical description: An elevated erythematous lesion with multiple pin-point blood vessels (strawberry lesion) is seen.

Histological description: Histopathology demonstrates a sharp transition from normal to acanthotic epithelium. The involved epithelium is markedly acanthotic and loss of polarity is noted. Other features may include solar elastosis of the stroma and mitotic figures (not shown).

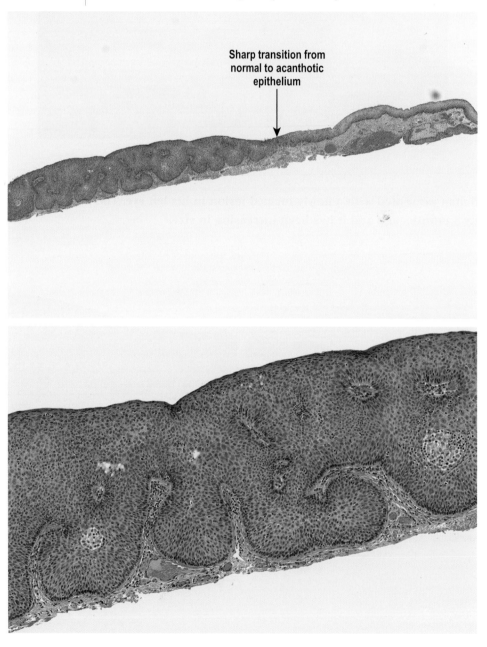

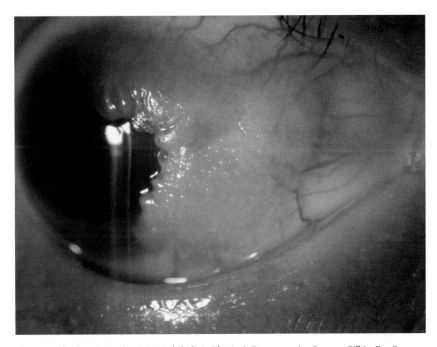

Courtesy of Robert J. Peralta, MD Ophthalmic Plastic & Reconstructive Surgery, Silkiss Eye Surgery.

The patient is a 68-year-old man with a 4-month history of a rapidly growing conjunctival lesion.

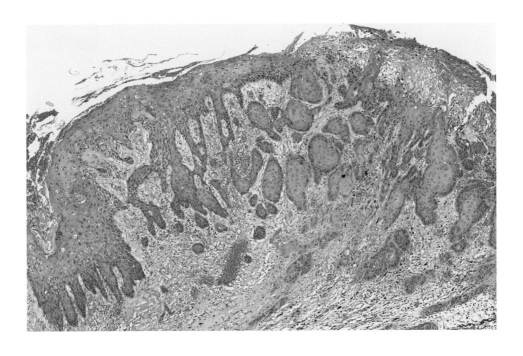

Diagnosis: Invasive conjunctival squamous cell carcinoma.

Clinical description: Anterior segment examination reveals an elevated lesion with a large feeder vessel. The lesion is arising from the conjunctiva and encroaching upon the cornea.

Histological description: There is a loss of polarity in the epithelium with marked atypia and pleomorphism. Nests of malignant squamous cells arising from the surface epithelium infiltrate the stroma (asterisks).

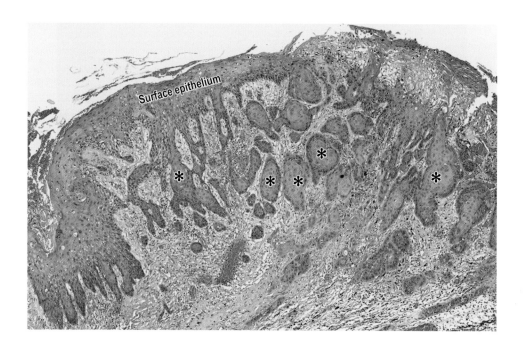

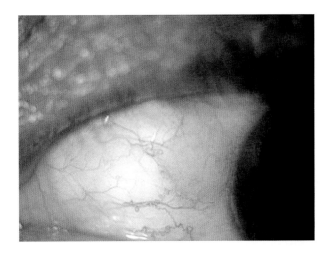

A 57-year-old man presented with conjunctival lesions of an unknown duration. He later underwent excision of the conjunctival lesions.

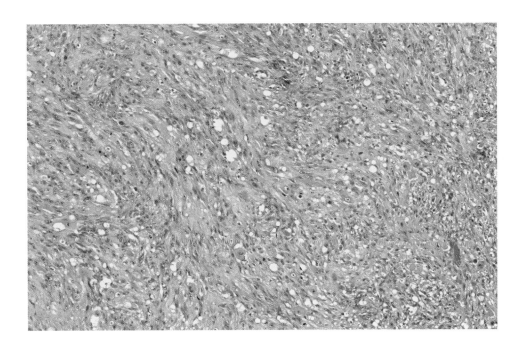

Diagnosis: Conjunctival fibrous histiocytoma.

Clinical description: Clinical examination reveals a red, elevated conjunctival lesion.

Histological description: Densely packed sheets of fibroblasts in a collagenous matrix are seen in a storiform pattern. Vacuolated histiocytes are noted in between the fibroblasts.

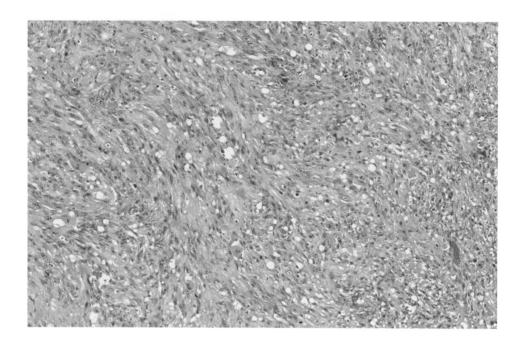

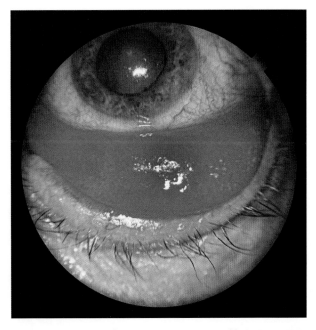

Printed with permission from Lee V., Azari A.A., Nehls S., Potter H.D., Albert D.A. Leiomyoma of the Lower Eyelid. JAMA Ophthalmology 2013; 131(8):1085.

A 55-year-old woman presented with eyelid swelling associated with irritation, excessive tearing, and mattering for over 1 month.

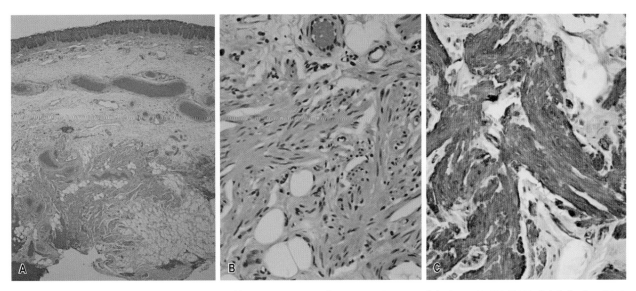

Printed with permission from Lee V., Azari A.A., Nehls S., Potter H.D., Albert D.A. Leiomyoma of the Lower Eyelid. JAMA Ophthalmology 2013; 131(8):1085.

Diagnosis: Leiomyoma of the conjunctiva.

Clinical description: Slit-lamp examination reveals an extensive red, elevated conjunctival lesion.

Histological description: (A) Histopathological evaluation demonstrates conjunctival tissue with an area of smooth muscle bundles. Higher magnification demonstrates fascicles composed of fusiform cells with cigar-shaped end nuclei (B). Cytoplasmic staining with muscle-specific actin stain is observed (C).

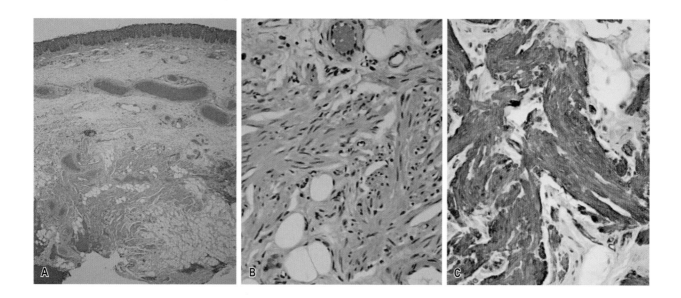

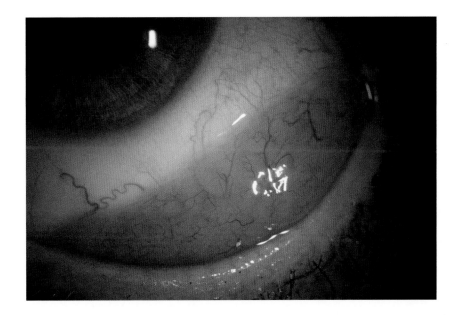

A 63-year-old man presented with a rapidly growing conjunctival mass. The conjunctival mass was removed and submitted for histopathological evaluation.

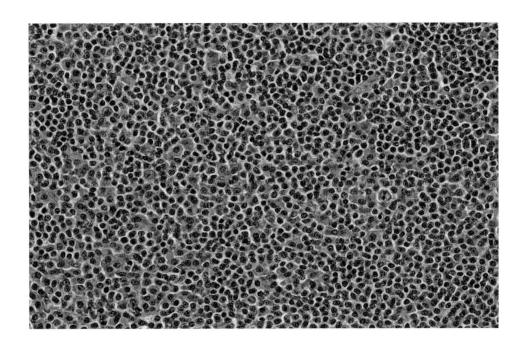

Diagnosis: Conjunctival mucosa-associated lymphoid tissue-type (MALT-type) lymphoma.

Clinical description: Clinical examination reveals a red, elevated conjunctival lesion with classic "salmon patch" appearance.

Histological description: Histopathological examination reveals proliferation of lymphocytes arranged in sheets.

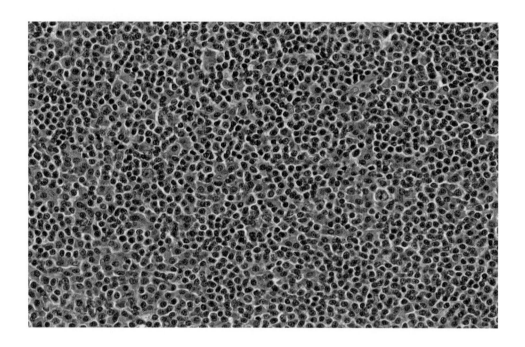

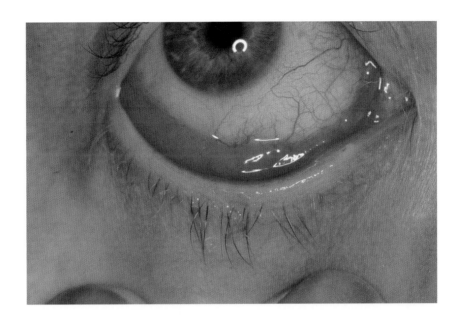

A 66-year-old woman presented with fullness under her right lower eyelid. She later underwent an excisional conjunctival biopsy.

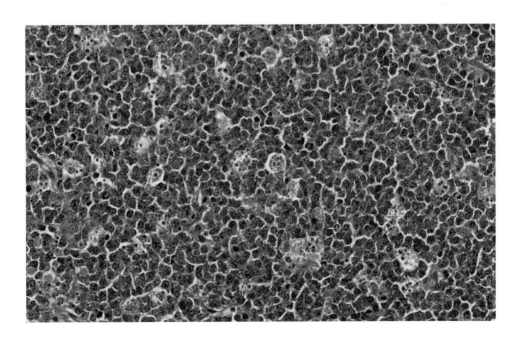

Diagnosis: Burkitt's lymphoma.

Clinical description: Clinical examination reveals a "salmon-patch" conjunctival lesion in the left lower fornix in this patient.

Histological description: Histopathology reveals tissue infiltrated with sheets of lymphocytes with presence of many tingible body macrophages. Tingible body macrophages are demonstrated with arrows. Note the "starry sky" appearance. Immunohistochemical staining confirmed the diagnosis of Burkitt's lymphoma.

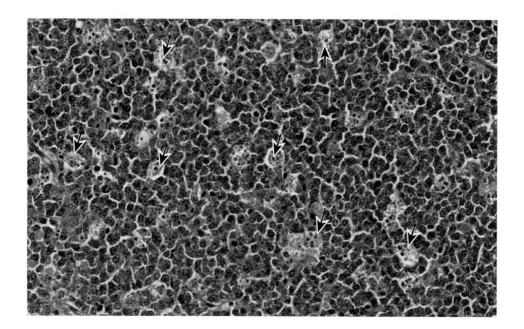

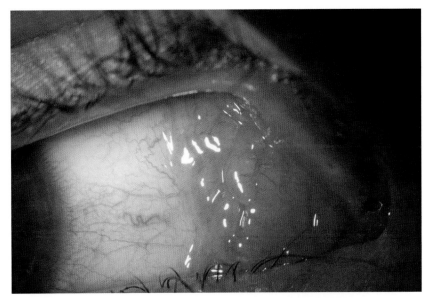

Courtesy of Sarah M. Nehls, M.D. University of Wisconsin-Madison.

A 42-year-old woman presented with foreign body sensation and a conjunctival mass for the past 6 months.

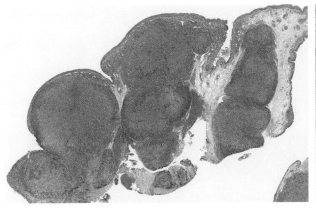 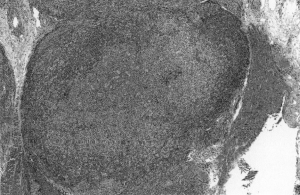

Diagnosis: Benign reactive lymphoid hyperplasia (BRLH).

Clinical description: Slit-limp examination shows a multilobulated red elevated conjunctival lesion.

Histological description: Histopathology demonstrates tissue with a nonkeratinized stratified squamous surface epithelium overlying multiple lymphoid follicles (asterisks). The follicles are composed of a germinal center and a mantle zone surrounding them. The follicular centers contain cleaved and noncleaved medium sized lymphoid cells with mitotic figures and tingible body macrophages (arrowheads).

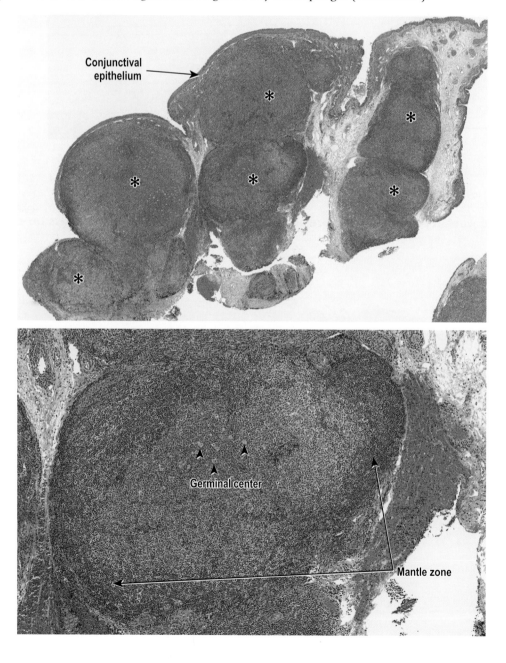

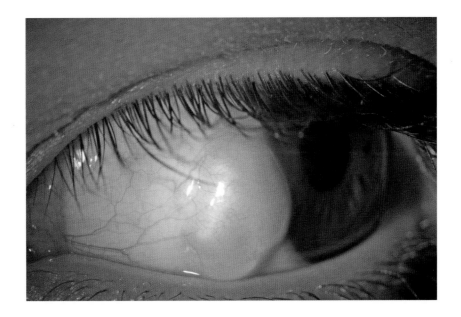

A 26-year-old woman presented with ocular irritation and foreign body sensation. She underwent excisional biopsy of the conjunctival lesion shown above.

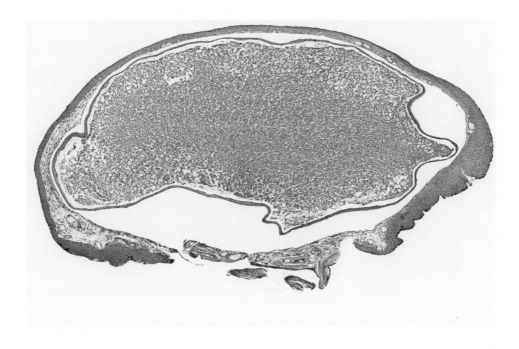

Diagnosis: Conjunctival inclusion cyst.

Clinical description: An elevated, well-circumscribed, fluid-filled conjunctival mass is seen.

Histological description: A large cystic space lined by nonkeratinized stratified squamous epithelium is seen within the conjunctival stroma. The cystic space is filled with exudative material.

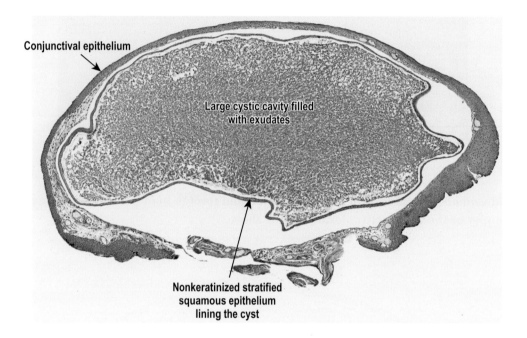

Conjunctival epithelium

Large cystic cavity filled with exudates

Nonkeratinized stratified squamous epithelium lining the cyst

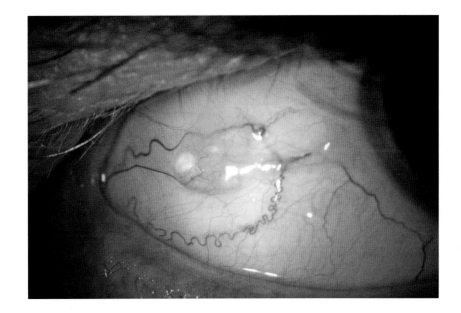

A 43-year-old woman presented with ocular irritation for the past 4 months. She later underwent an excisional biopsy of the conjunctival lesion.

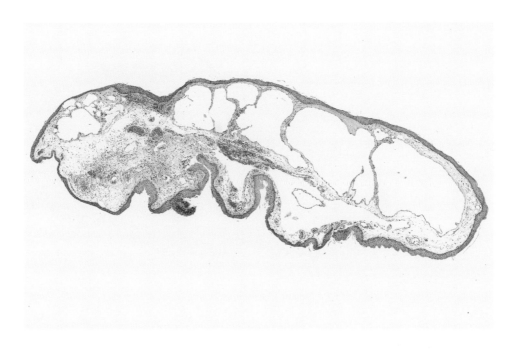

Diagnosis: Conjunctival lymphangiectasia.

Clinical description: Clinical examination demonstrates thin-walled translucent cystic spaces on the temporal aspect of the bulbar conjunctiva.

Histological description: Histopathological examination reveals conjunctiva with multi-loculated cystic spaces (asterisks) in the substantia propria (stroma) lined by thin walls and flattened endothelial cells.

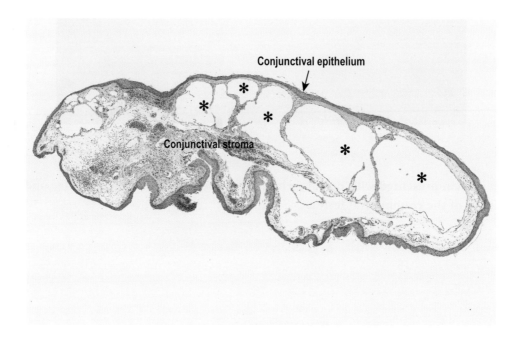

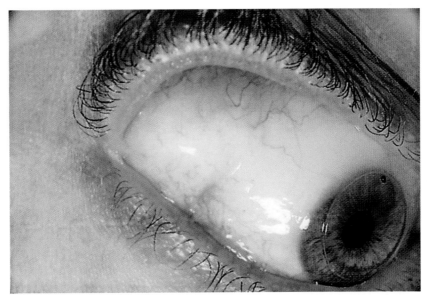

A 43-year-old woman presented with a mass under her right upper eyelid. The mass was excised and evaluated histopathologically.

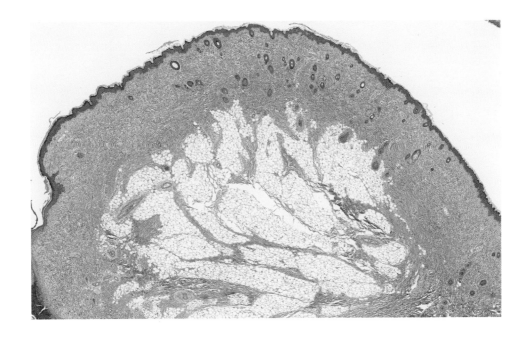

Diagnosis: Lipodermoid.

Clinical description: Slit-lamp examination reveals a fatty, elevated, supratemporal subconjunctival lesion. Also noted is the rigid gas-permeable contact lens worn by the patient.

Histological description: Histopathology reveals tissue covered by stratified squamous epithelium. The stroma is collagenous and contains aggregates of lipid cells.

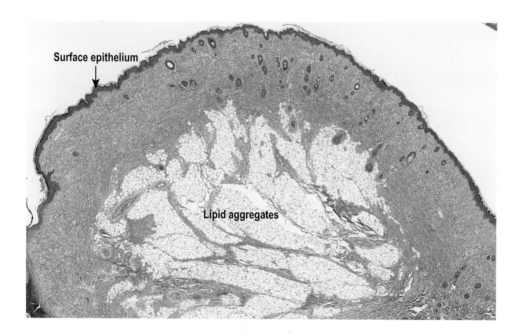

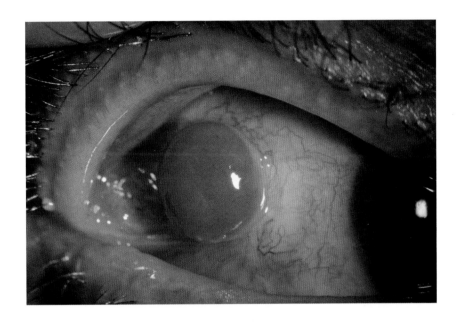

A 22-year-old man with a past ocular history significant for conjunctival laceration presented with a red exuberant conjunctival mass.

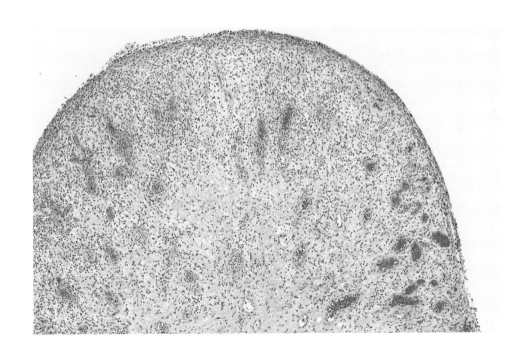

Diagnosis: Pyogenic granuloma.

Clinical description: A well-circumscribed, red, elevated lesion with a smooth surface arising from the bulbar conjunctiva.

Histological description: The histopathology demonstrates an exuberant tissue with an edematous stroma. Acute and chronic nongranulomatous inflammation and radiating blood vessels are present.

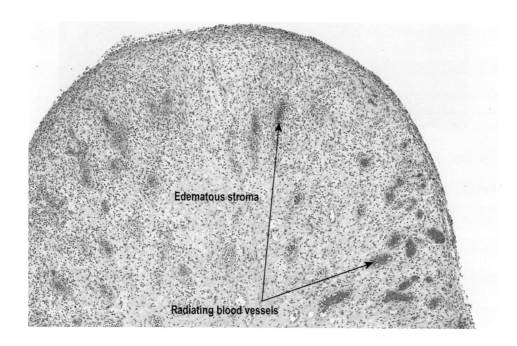

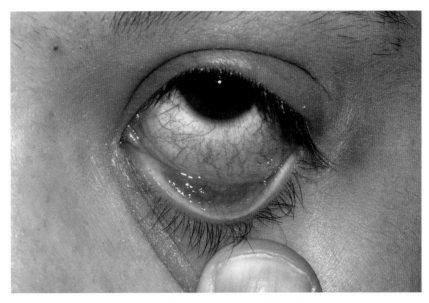

From Albert, Daniel M., Miller, Joan W., Azar, Dimitri T., and Blodi, Barbara A. (eds). 2008. Albert & Jakobiec's Principles and Practice of Ophthalmology, 3rd ed. Philadelphia: Copyright Elsevier 2008.

A 23-year-old man presented with discharge from his left eye for the past 3 days.

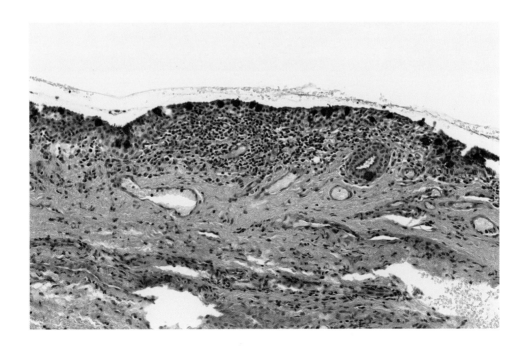

Diagnosis: Bacterial conjunctivitis.

Clinical description: Clinical examination demonstrates conjunctival redness, hyperemia, and mild discharge.

Histological description: Histological examination reveals tissue lined by goblet-cell-containing, nonkeratinized epithelium. The conjunctival stroma is infiltrated with lymphocytes and plasma cells (circle).

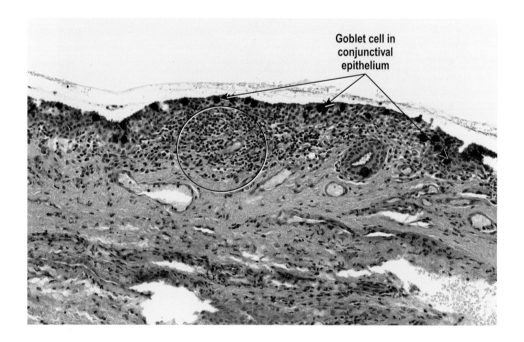

Goblet cell in
conjunctival
epithelium

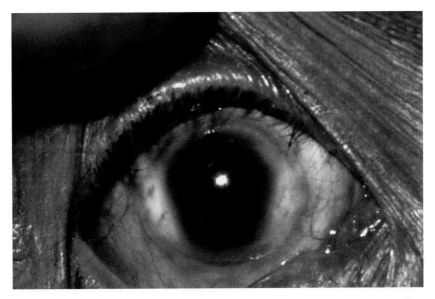

From Albert, Daniel M., Miller, Joan W., Azar, Dimitri T., and Blodi, Barbara A. (eds). 2008. Albert & Jakobiec's Principles and Practice of Ophthalmology, 3rd ed. Philadelphia: Copyright Elsevier 2008.

A 46-year-old patient presented with ocular pain and redness.

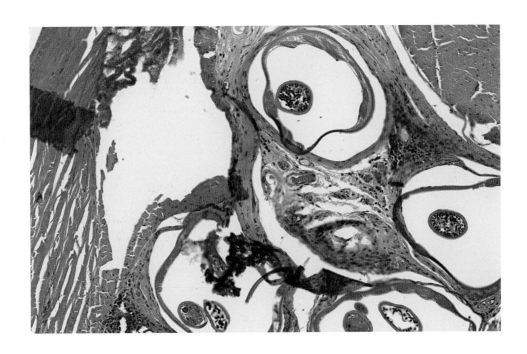

Diagnosis: Onchocerciasis.

Clinical description: Slit-lamp examination reveals marked conjunctival redness and chemosis.

Histological description: Histopathological examination reveals a cross-sectional view of the *Onchocerca volvulus*.

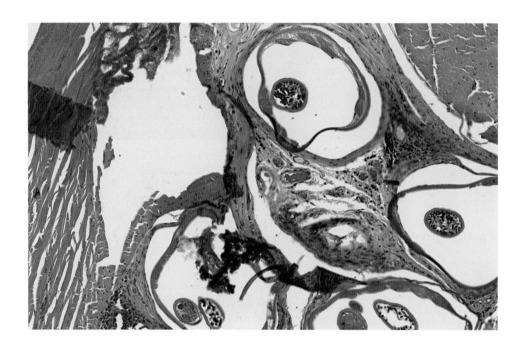

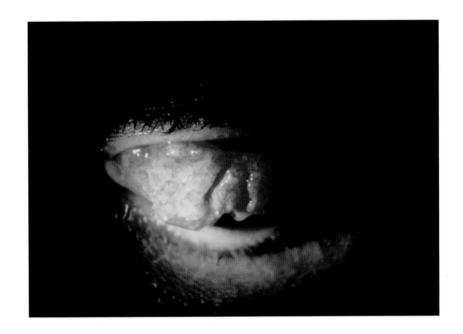

A 10-year-old healthy boy presented with ocular irritation and a large eyelid lesion.

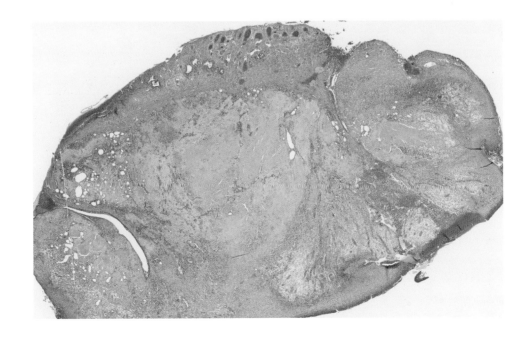

Diagnosis: Ligneous conjunctivitis.

Clinical description: Slit-lamp examination shows a solid "woody" lesion in the superior tarsal conjunctiva.

Histological description: Histopathology demonstrates amorphous eosinophilic substance within the conjunctival stroma. The conjunctival surface epithelium is not present in this section.

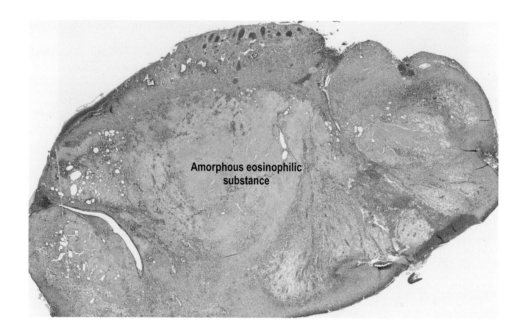

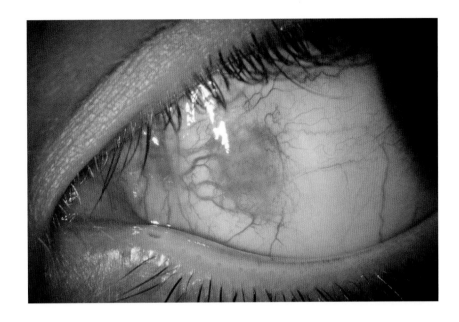

A 32-year-old African American woman with a history of shortness of breath presented with a conjunctival lesion, as shown above.

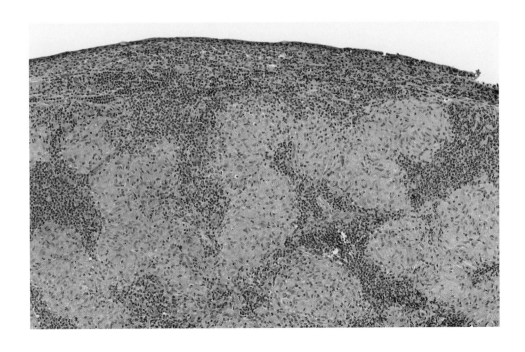

Diagnosis: Conjunctival sarcoidosis.

Clinical description: Slit-lamp examination reveals a red, elevated subconjunctival lesion in the nasal bulbar conjunctiva of the right eye.

Histological description: Histopathology demonstrates diffuse infiltration of the conjunctival stroma by sheets of mononuclear inflammatory cells and tubercles of epithelioid and giant cells. No significant caseation is present.

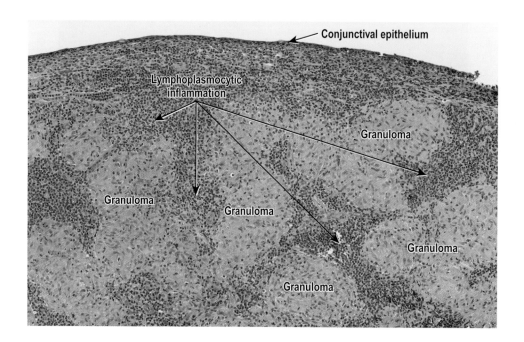

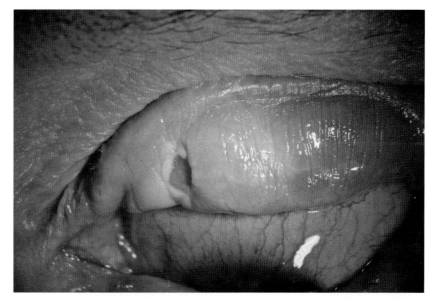

Courtesy of Heather D. Potter, M.D. University of Wisconsin-Madison.

The patient is a 57-year-old woman with a history of eye rubbing. She underwent an excisional biopsy of the left tarsal conjunctiva.

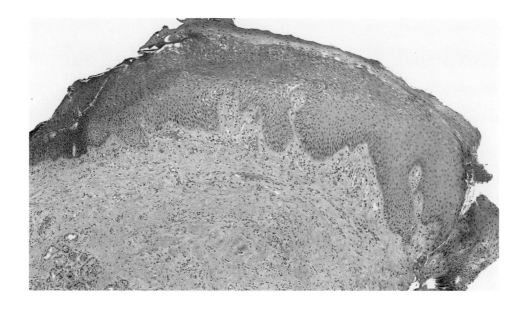

Diagnosis: Lichen simplex chronicus.

Clinical description: Clinical examination after the eversion of the left upper eyelid demonstrates thickening and laceration of the tarsal conjunctiva.

Histological description: Histopathology demonstrates tissue lined by metaplastic conjunctiva showing squamatization composed of uniform keratinocytes with compact ortho- and parakeratosis. A mild lymphocytic infiltrate is seen in the substantia propria. There is loss of collagen density in the tarsus. Glandular structures are also noted in the substantia propria (asterisk).

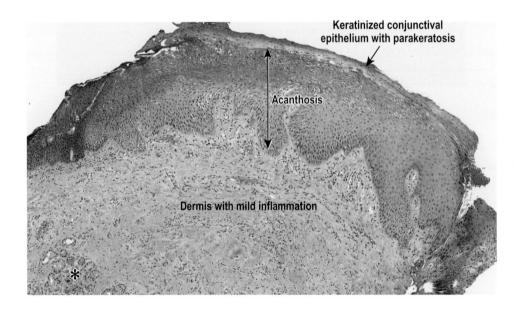

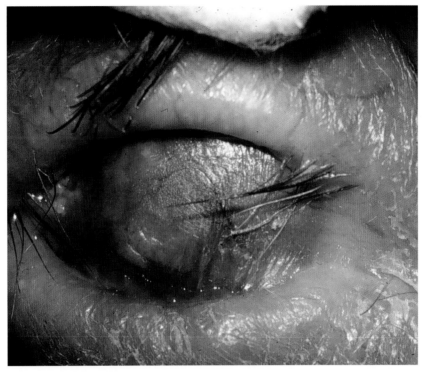

Courtesy of Neal P. Barney, M.D. University of Wisconsin-Madison.

A 65-year-old woman with chronic ocular discomfort and decreased vision underwent a conjunctival biopsy.

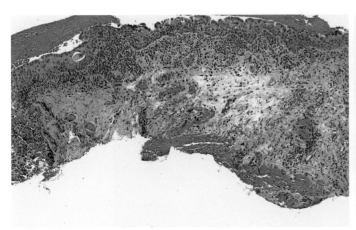 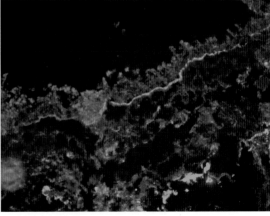

Diagnosis: Ocular cicatricial pemphigoid.

Clinical description: The clinical image demonstrates corneal opacity, trichiasis, madarosis, and symblepharon formation.

Histological description: Histopathology demonstrates marked conjunctival inflammation (top). Immunohistochemistry demonstrates a linear band of IgG in the conjunctival epithelial basement membrane.

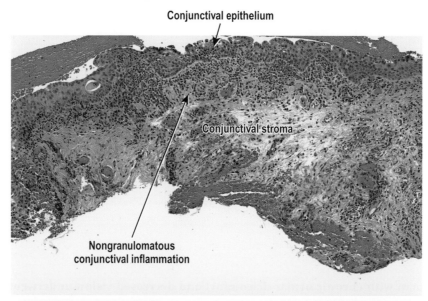

Conjunctival epithelium

Conjunctival stroma

Nongranulomatous
conjunctival inflammation

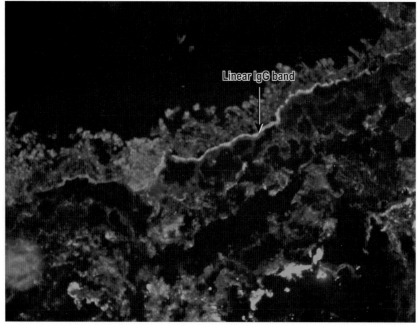

Linear IgG band

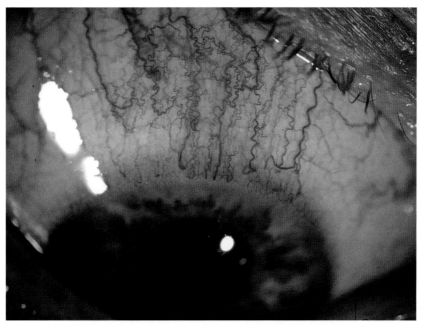

Courtesy of Neal P. Barney, M.D. University of Wisconsin-Madison.

A 54-year-old woman presented with dry eyes and foreign body sensation. The patient had been using artificial tears with no relief. She underwent excision of the superior bulbar conjunctiva.

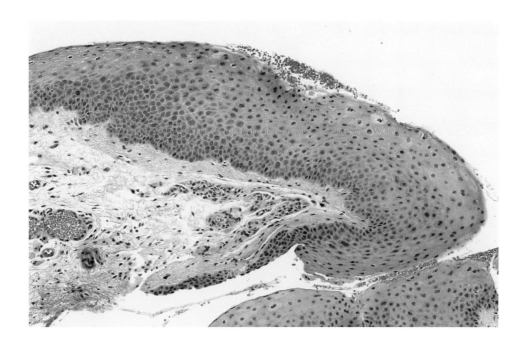

Diagnosis: Superior limbic keratoconjunctivitis.

Clinical description: Marked vascular dilation, hyperemia, and thickening is seen in the superior bulbar conjunctiva.

Histological description: The specimen consists of conjunctival tissue showing areas of epithelial thickening, degeneration, and complete loss of goblet cells. Nuclear pseudoinclusions and abnormal aggregations of chromatin are seen within many cells. A nongranulomatous mixed inflammatory infiltrate is seen within the substantia propria and epithelium.

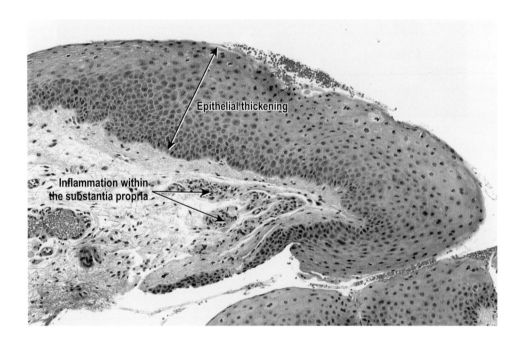

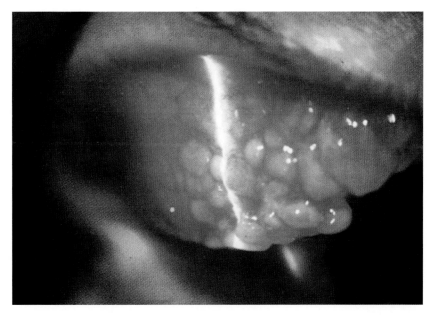

From Albert, Daniel M., Miller, Joan W., Azar, Dimitri T., and Blodi, Barbara A. (eds). 2008. Albert & Jakobiec's Principles and Practice of Ophthalmology, 3rd ed. Philadelphia: Copyright Elsevier 2008.

A 6-year-old boy presented with bilateral itching of the eyes and foreign body sensation. A few similar episodes in the past were treated with topical steroids.

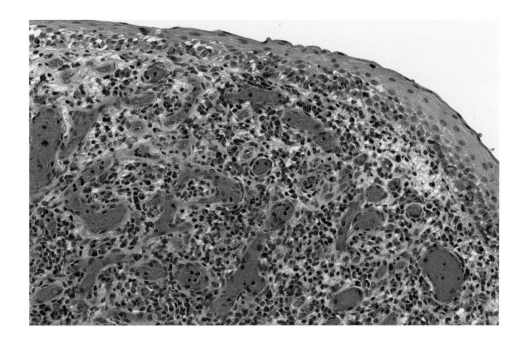

Diagnosis: Vernal keratoconjunctivitis.

Clinical description: The clinical examination demonstrates presence of giant papillae on the tarsal conjunctiva when the upper eyelid is everted.

Histological description: Histopathological examination reveals conjunctiva with stratified squamous epithelium. The epithelium shows focal areas with lymphocytic and eosinophilic infiltration. Marked diffuse eosinophilic infiltration (some are shown with arrows) as well as chronic lymphoplasmacytic inflammation is seen within a vascular (asterisks) stroma.

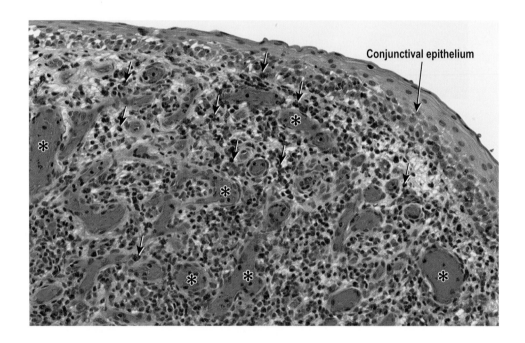

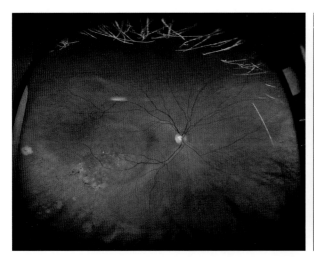 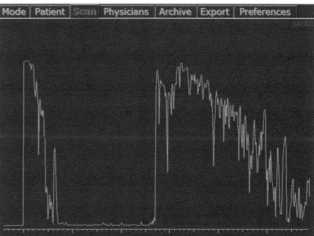

A 48-year-old woman presented with decreased vision over the past 8 months. The fundus image and ultrasound findings are depicted above.

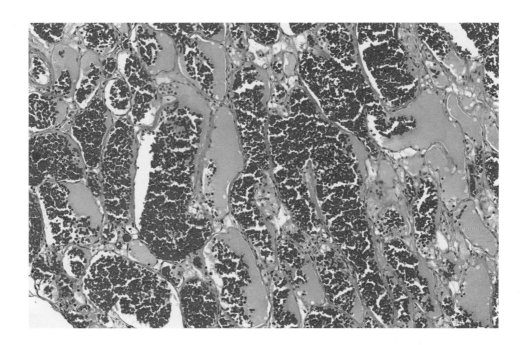

Diagnosis: Choroidal hemangioma.

Clinical description: An elevated subretinal lesion demonstrating high internal reflectivity on A-scan is seen.

Histological description: Histopathology reveals dilated vascular channels that are lined by a single layer of flat endothelium. The vascular channels are filled with red blood cells.

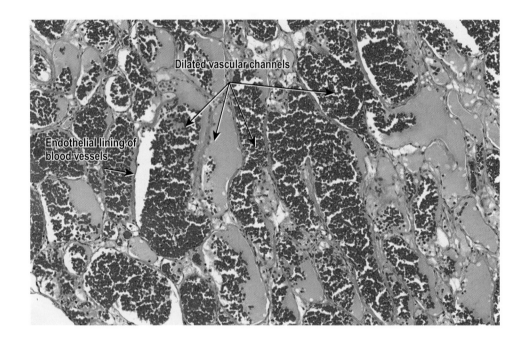

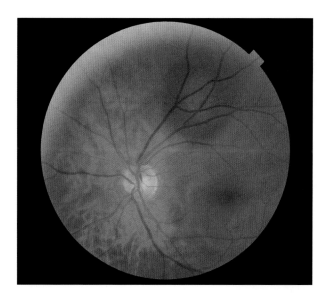

A 28-year-old woman presented with a pigmented choroidal mass.

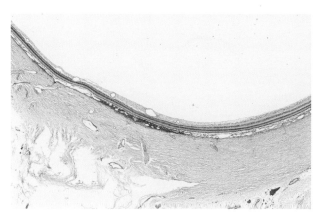 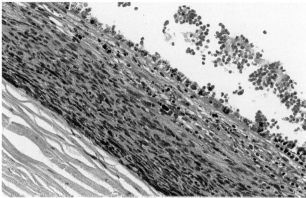

Diagnosis: Choroidal nevus.

Clinical description: Dilated fundus examination demonstrates a darkly pigmented choroidal mass.

Histological description: Proliferation of melanocytic cells is seen within the choroid. The cells appear benign and mitotic figures are not present.

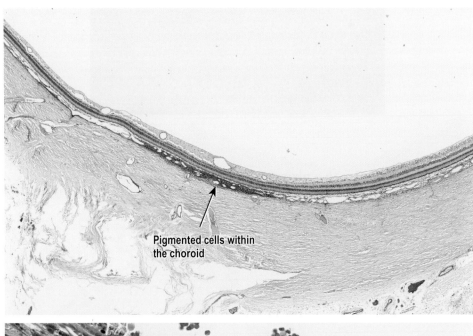

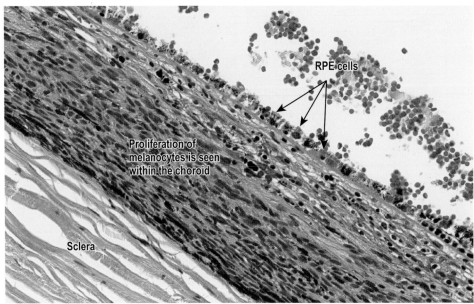

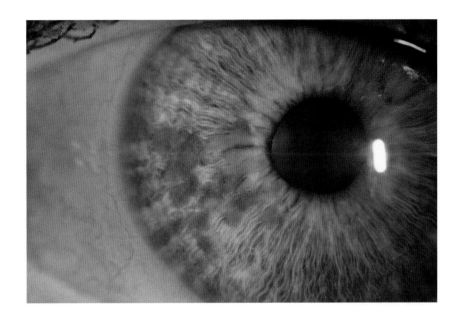

A 47-year-old woman presented with multiple iris lesions. No iris lesions were present in her other eye.

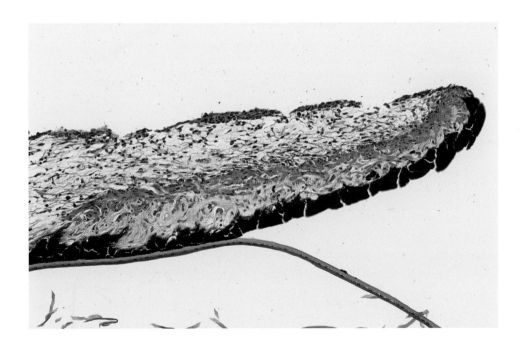

Diagnosis: Iris nevi.

Clinical description: Elevated, nodular pigmented lesions are seen.

Histological description: Multiple areas of melanocytic proliferation consistent with nevi are seen on the iris surface (arrows).

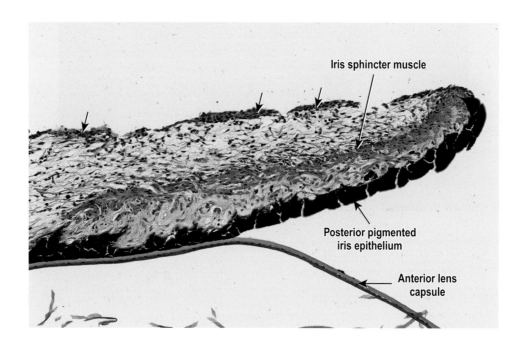

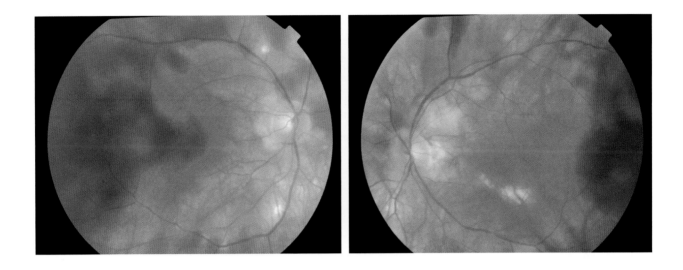

A 70-year-old woman under treatment for ovarian carcinoma presented with bilateral decreased vision for the past 2 months.

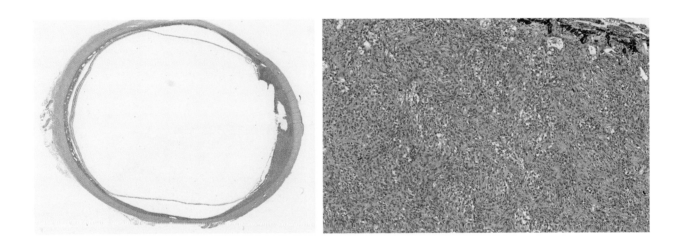

Diagnosis: Bilateral diffuse uveal melanocytic proliferation (BDUMP), a paraneoplastic syndrome.

Clinical description: The fundus examination reveals bilateral patchy pigmented subretinal lesions.

Histological description: Histopathological examination of collette following enucleation at autopsy reveals diffuse thickening of the choroid and increase in uveal melanocytic cells.

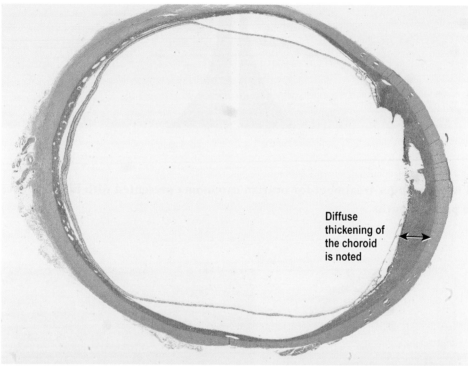

Diffuse thickening of the choroid is noted

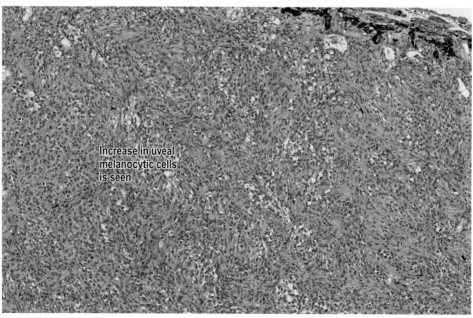

Increase in uveal melanocytic cells is seen

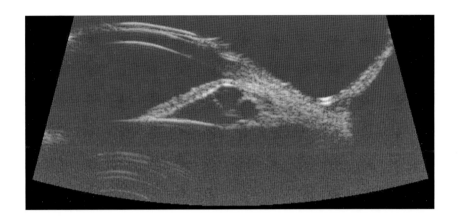

A 67-year-old man presented with a new iris lesion, as shown above.

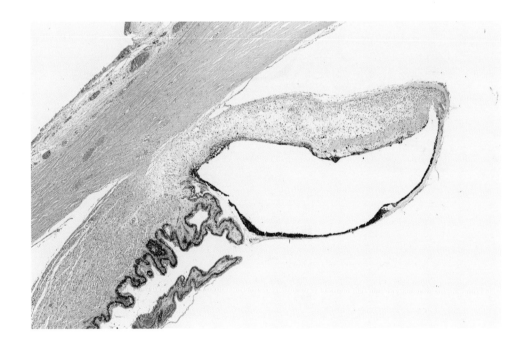

Diagnosis: Iris cyst.

Clinical description: Ultrasound demonstrates a posterior cystic iris lesion.

Histological description: Histopathology reveals a large cystic cavity within the posterior pigmented iris epithelium.

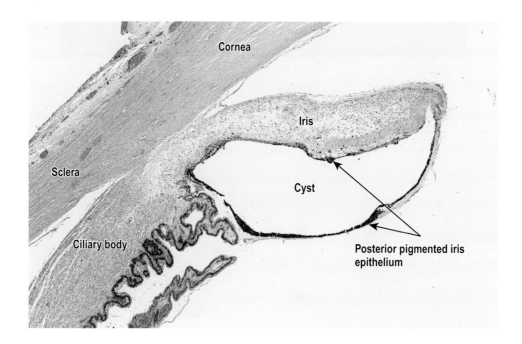

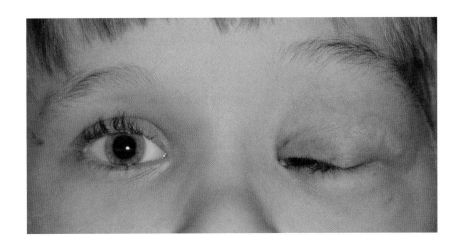

An 8-year-old boy presented with the above eyelid deformity.

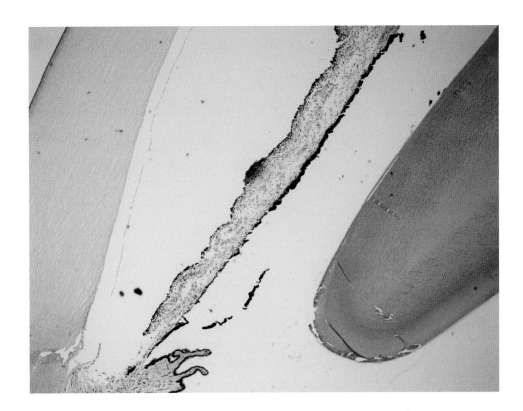

Diagnosis: Lisch nodule in neurofibromatosis type 1.

Clinical description: Clinical examination reveals an "S-shaped" eyelid deformity.

Histological description: Nodular aggregates of melanocytes, consistent with a Lisch nodule, are seen in the anterior iris.

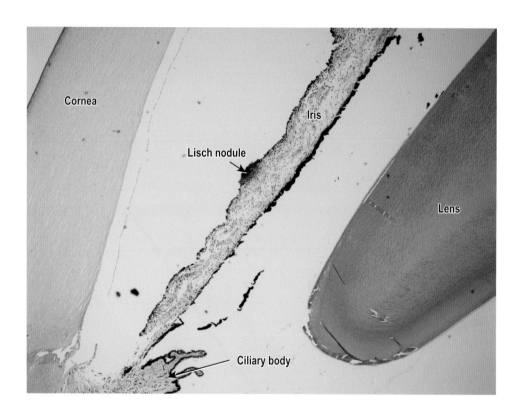

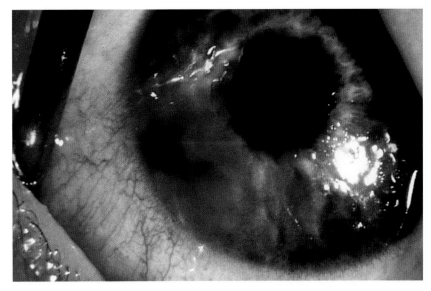

A 5-year-old boy presented with an iris lesion, present for the past 8 months.

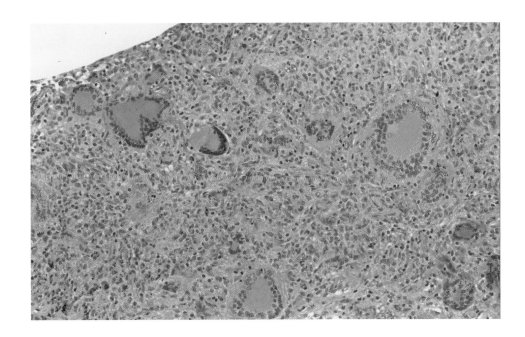

Diagnosis: Juvenile xanthogranuloma presenting with an iris mass.

Clinical description: Slit-lamp examination demonstrates a localized iris plaque.

Histological description: Histopathology reveals tissue infiltrated with inflammatory cells and Touton multinucleated giant cells (arrows).

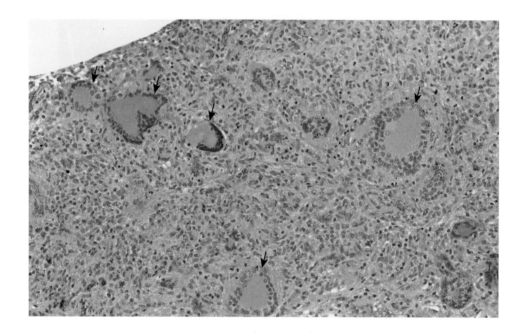

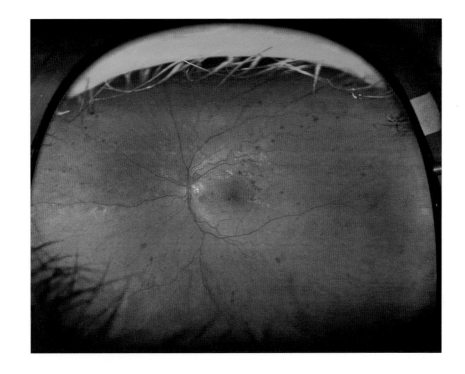

A 66-year-old man with insulin dependent diabetes mellitus presented with blurry vision.

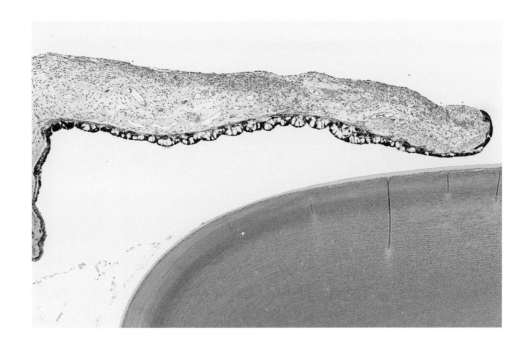

Diagnosis: Lacy iris vacuolization in a patient with diabetes mellitus.

Clinical description: The dilated fundus examination shows numerous retinal hemorrhages as well as neovascularization at the head of the optic nerve.

Histological description: Histopathology reveals lacy vacuolization (arrows) of the posterior pigmented iris epithelium.

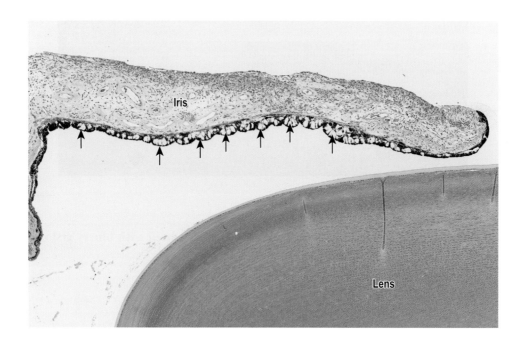

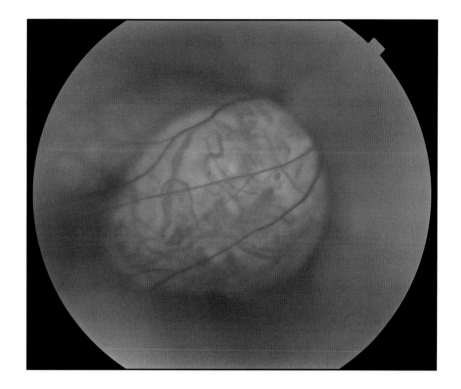

A 59-year-old man presented with gradual loss of vision. He later underwent enucleation.

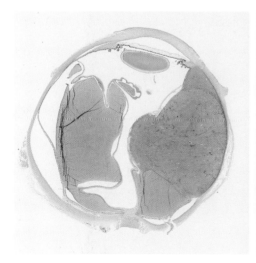

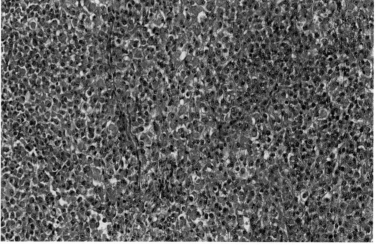

Diagnosis: Choroidal melanoma (epithelioid type).

Clinical description: A large elevated choroidal lesion is seen on dilated fundus examination.

Histological description: A mushroom-shaped mass is seen arising from the choroid. The tumor cells demonstrate considerable cytoplasm (arrows) with a large nucleus and prominent nucleoli (arrowheads). The cell boundaries are distinct, and there is lack of cohesion between the tumor cells. An exudative retinal detachment is also present (asterisk).

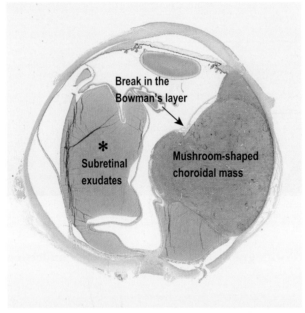

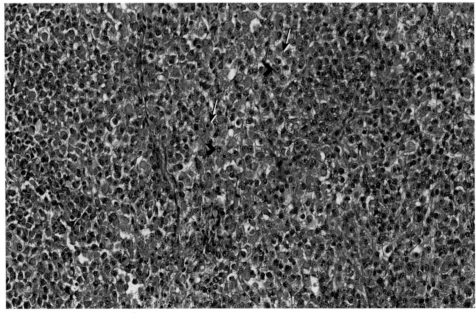

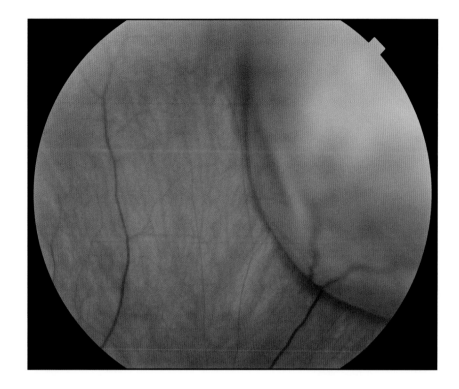

A 58-year-old woman presented with loss of vision. The clinical examination findings are depicted above. She later underwent an enucleation.

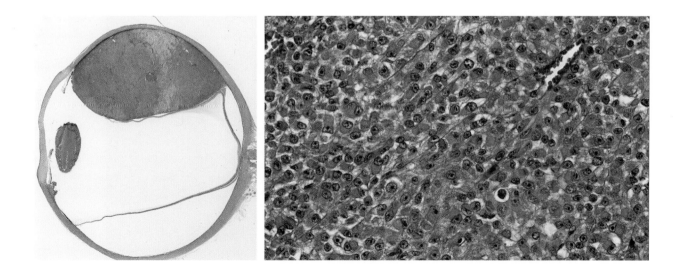

Diagnosis: Ciliary body melanoma (epithelioid type).

Clinical description: A large elevated ciliary body mass on dilated fundus examination is seen.

Histological description: Histopathology demonstrates a large mass proliferating from the ciliary body (top). Large epithelioid cells with abundant cytoplasm, large nuclei, and distinct nucleoli are seen. The cell borders are distinct and the cells are discohesive.

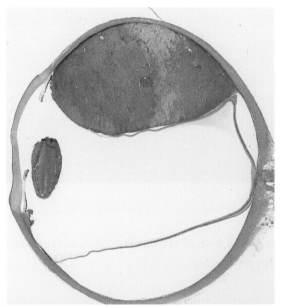

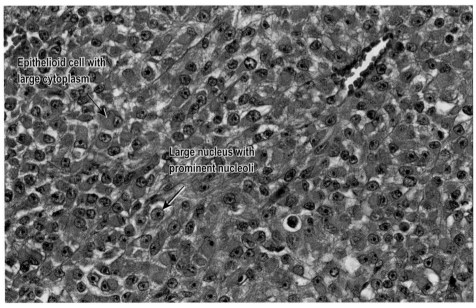

Epithelioid cell with large cytoplasm

Large nucleus with prominent nucleoli

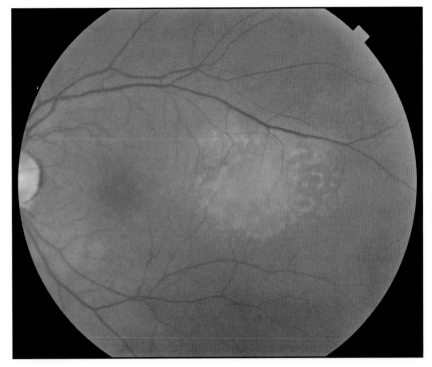

Courtesy of Justin Gottlieb, MD, University of Wisconsin-Madison.

A 37-year-old woman presented with the above incidental finding.

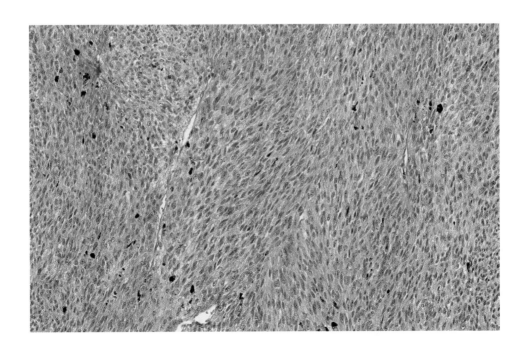

Diagnosis: Spindle cell melanoma.

Clinical description: Dilated fundus examination shows a large elevated pigmented choroidal mass in the posterior pole.

Histological description: Proliferation of spindle cells with elongated nucleus and inconspicuous nucleoli. Cell boundaries are indistinct with a syncytial pattern.

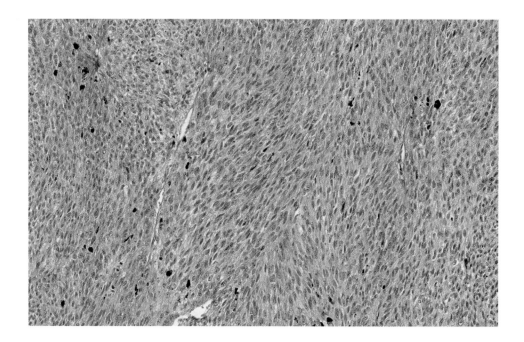

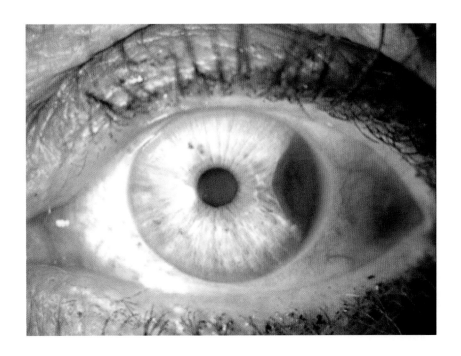

A 58-year-old woman presented with a pigmented iris lesion in her left eye.

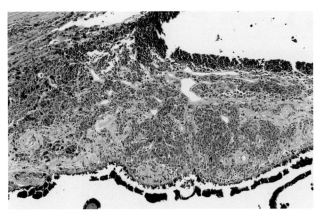 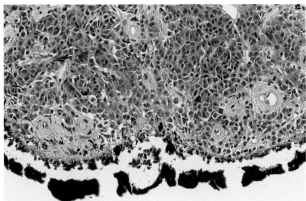

Diagnosis: Iris melanoma.

Clinical description: A slightly elevated pigmented iris lesion is noted on the slit-lamp examination.

Histological description: Histopathology reveals infiltration of the iris tissue with atypical melanocytes. The cells demonstrate a large nuclear to cytoplasmic ratio.

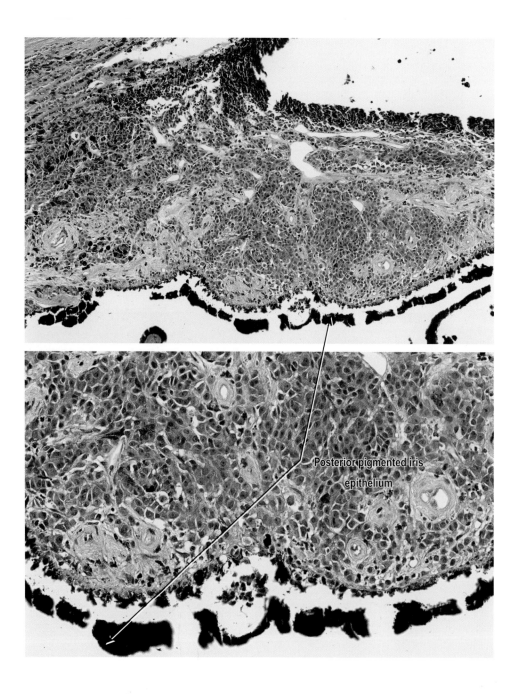

Posterior pigmented iris epithelium

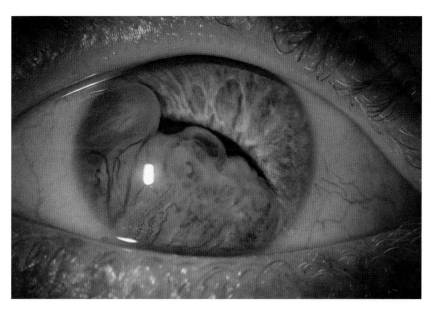

Printed with permission from Lewis, David A., Nehls, Sarah, et al. Ciliary Body Medulloepithelioma in a 10-Year-Old Boy. Arch Ophthalmol. 2012 Jul;130(7):881.

A 10-year-old boy presented with decreased vision and an intraocular mass.

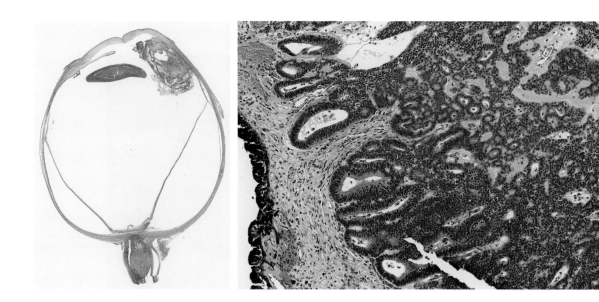

Diagnosis: Medulloepithelioma.

Clinical description: A cystic vascular nonpigmented mass is seen in the anterior chamber.

Histological description: Histopathological evaluation demonstrates cystic spaces filled with hyaluronic acid (asterisk) surrounded by primitive neuroepithelial cells arranged in sheets, cords, tubules, and rosette-like formations.

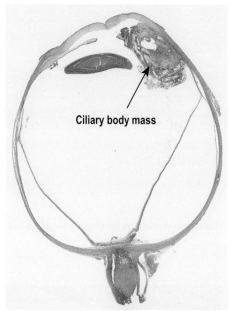

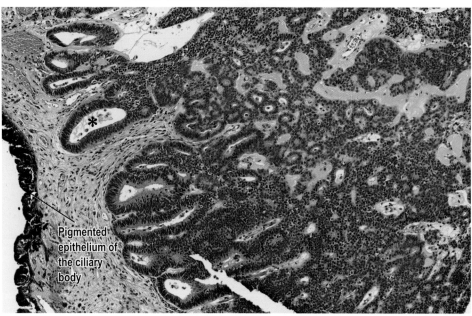

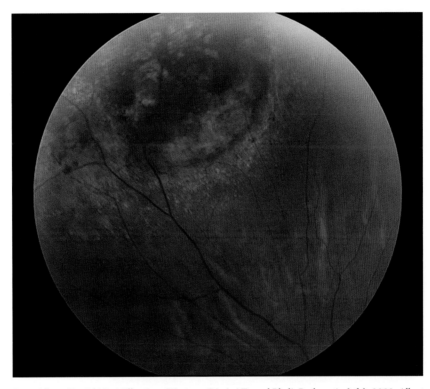

From Albert, Daniel M., Miller, Joan W., Azar, Dimitri T., and Blodi, Barbara A. (eds). 2008. Albert & Jakobiec's Principles and Practice of Ophthalmology, 3rd ed. Philadelphia: Copyright Elsevier 2008.

A 59-year-old woman with a history of choroidal melanoma treated with plaque therapy. She subsequently developed a blind painful eye with LP vision and the eye was enucleated.

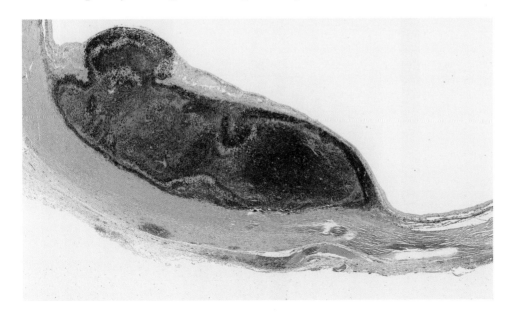

Diagnosis: Choroidal melanoma after plaque therapy.

Clinical description: Dilated fundus examination reveals a pigmented choroidal lesion surrounded by atrophic changes in the retina and choroid.

Histological description: A pigmented tumor is seen arising from the choroid and involving the retina. The tumor is highly necrotic and it is composed of epithelioid cells and pigment-laden macrophages. The retina overlying the tumor is severely atrophic. The sclera overlying the tumor shows areas of inflammation and fragmentation.

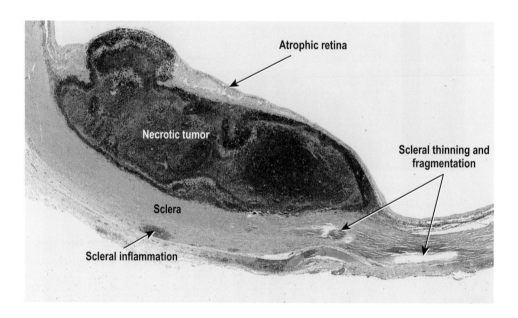

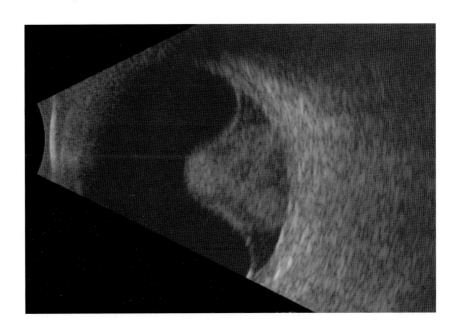

A 49-year-old man presented with decreased vision. A choroidal mass was noted on dilated fundus examination. The ultrasound findings are depicted above. He later underwent an enucleation.

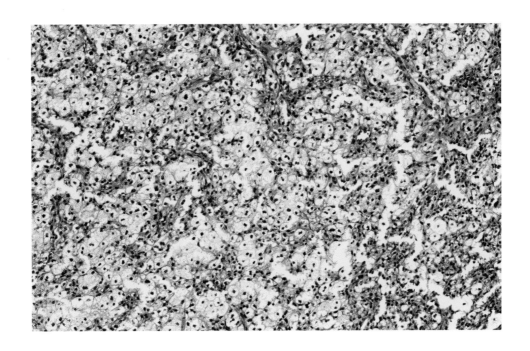

Diagnosis: Balloon cell melanoma.

Clinical description: Dilated fundus examination reveals an elevated dome-shaped choroidal mass with an overlying retinal detachment.

Histological description: Numerous balloon cells (arrows) exhibiting abundant clear cytoplasm are seen.

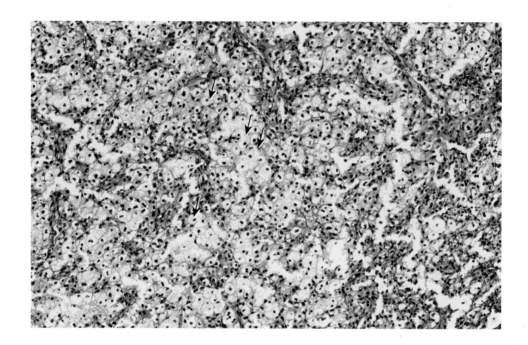

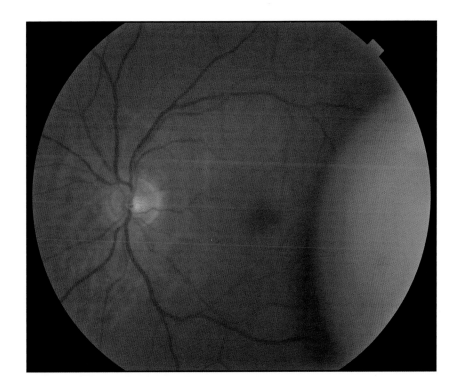

An 81-year-old man presented complaining of a gradual decrease in his peripheral vision.

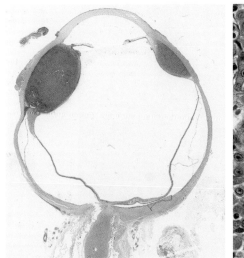

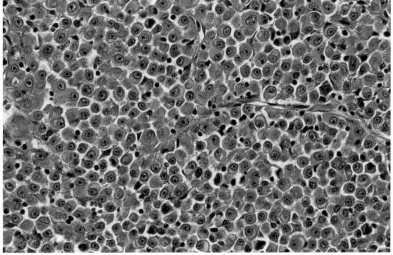

Diagnosis: Ring melanoma of the ciliary body (epithelioid type).

Clinical description: Dilated fundus examination reveals a large ciliary body mass.

Histological description: Histopathological examination demonstrates tumor arising from the ciliary body (top). Large epithelioid cells with abundant cytoplasm, large nuclei, and prominent nucleoli are seen. The cells have well-defined borders and they are discohesive.

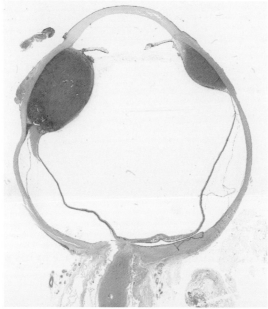

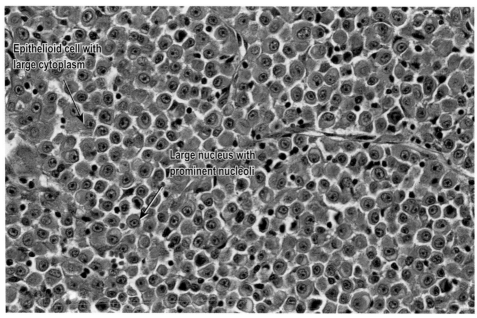

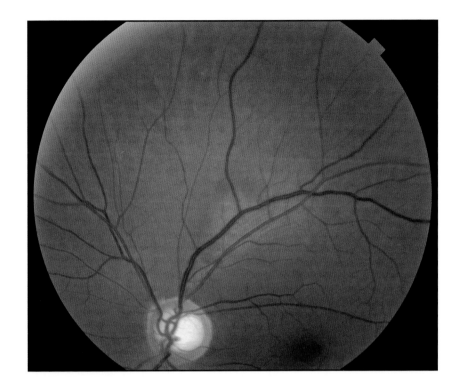

The patient is a 54-year-old man with a history of choroidal mass in his left eye. The patient's past medical history is significant for renal cell carcinoma.

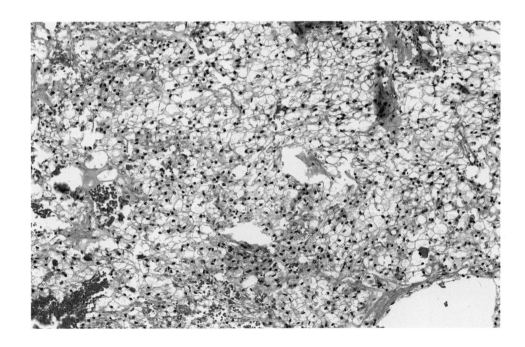

Diagnosis: Metastatic renal cell carcinoma to choroid.

Clinical description: The dilated fundus examination reveals an elevated choroidal mass superior to the optic nerve head.

Histological description: Histopathology reveals a tumor that is composed of rounded-to-polygonal-shaped cells with abundant clear cytoplasm (clear cells) (some of which are shown with arrows) consistent with renal cell carcinoma. The stroma of the tumor is highly vascular.

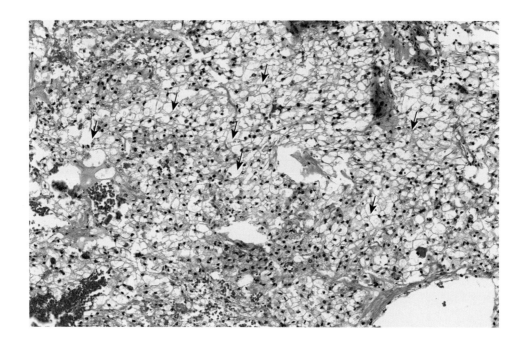

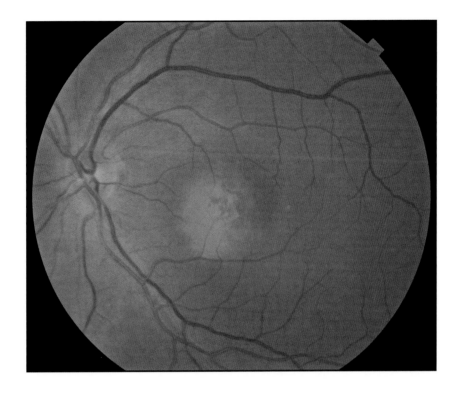

A 68-year-old woman with a history of breast cancer presented with loss of vision in her left eye.

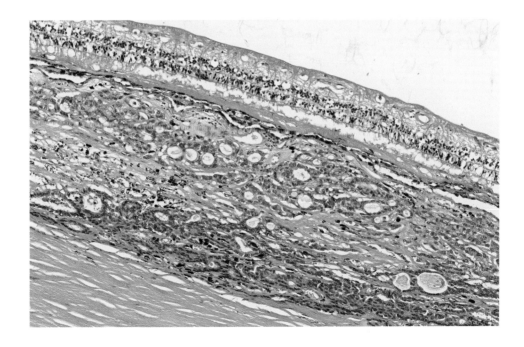

Diagnosis: Metastatic breast cancer to choroid.

Clinical description: Dilated fundus examination reveals a large elevated choroidal lesion within the center of the macula.

Histological description: Histopathology reveals the choroidal tissue infiltrated with epithelial cells, some exhibiting "Indian-file" arrangement (arrows). These cells are round with eosinophilic cytoplasm. Areas of duct formation are also seen (asterisks).

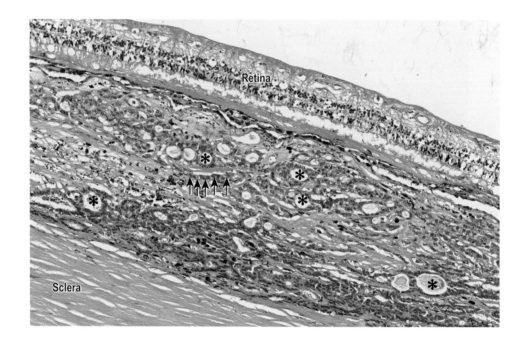

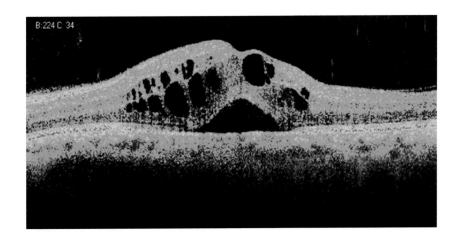

An 82-year-old man presented with decreased vision and the above OCT findings following a complicated cataract surgery.

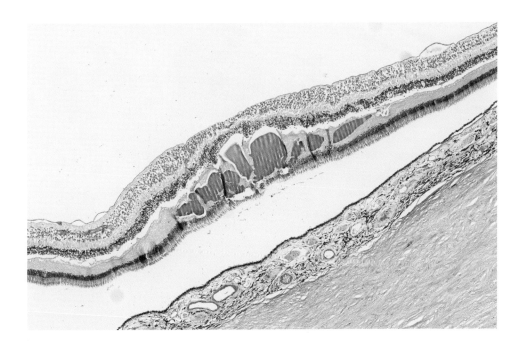

Diagnosis: Cystoid macular edema.

Clinical description: Large cystic cavities are seen within the outer plexiform layer.

Histological description: Large amounts of exudates are seen within the outer plexiform layer.

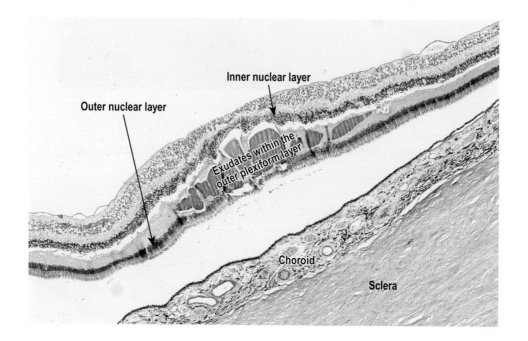

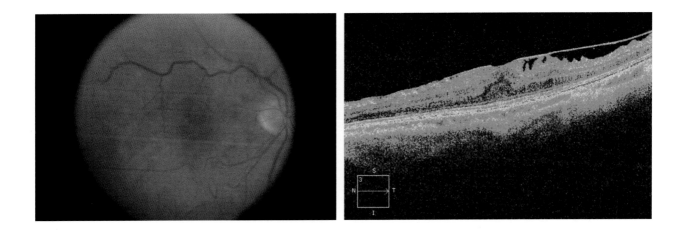

A 73-year-old man presented with decreased vision in his right eye. The fundus appearance and OCT findings are depicted above.

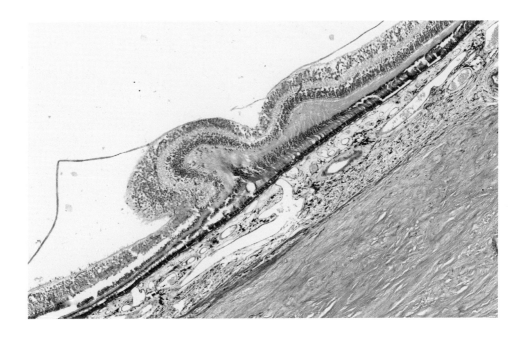

Diagnosis: Epiretinal membrane (macular pucker).

Clinical description: Fundus examination demonstrates macular puckering. OCT shows the well-delineated epiretinal membrane.

Histological description: Traction from the epiretinal membrane (ERM) has resulted in retinal folds.

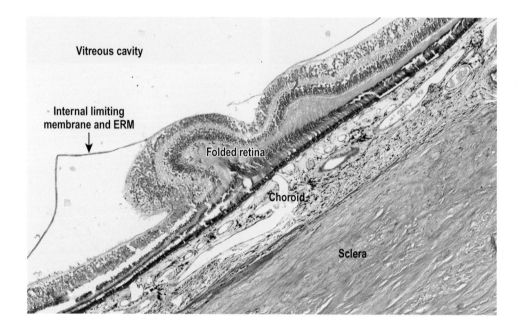

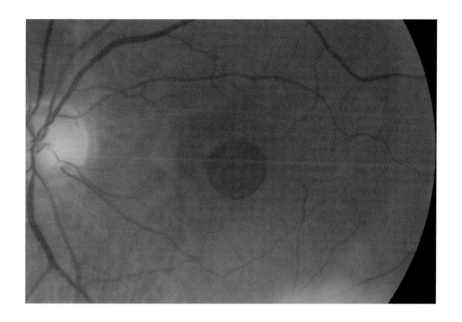

A 78-year-old woman presented with decreased vision in her left eye.

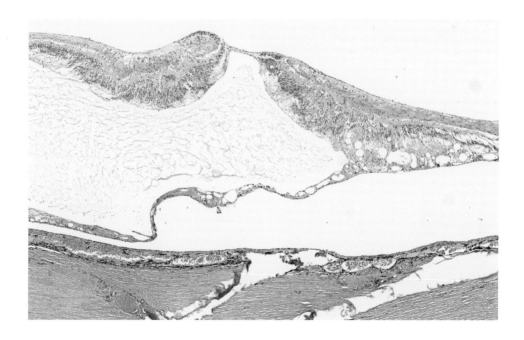

Diagnosis: Macular hole.

Clinical description: Dilated fundus examination reveals a round well-delineated macular hole.

Histological description: Histopathology is consistent with a macular hole.

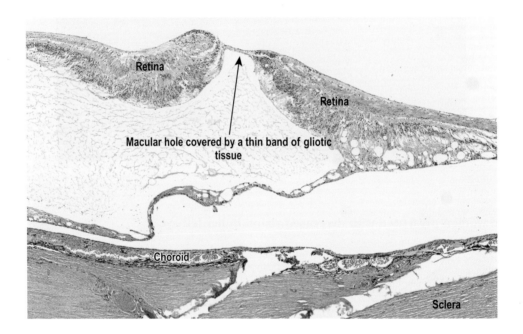

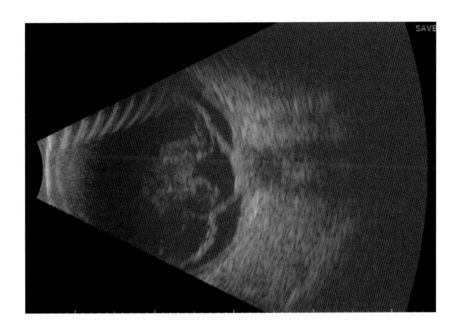

A 72-year-old man presented with loss of vision in his right eye. The ultrasound findings are depicted above. The eye later underwent an enucleation.

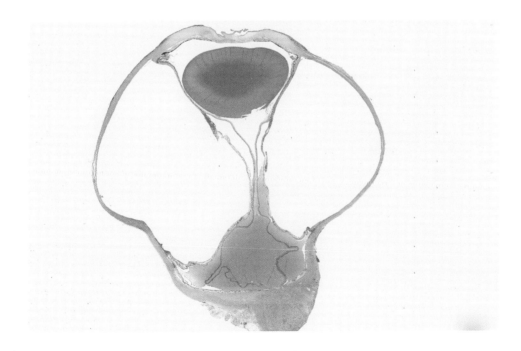

Diagnosis: Funnel-shaped retinal detachment.

Clinical description: Ultrasound reveals a funnel-shaped retinal detachment.

Histological description: A funnel-shaped retinal detachment is evident on histopathology. The retina remains attached to the optic nerve and ora serrata.

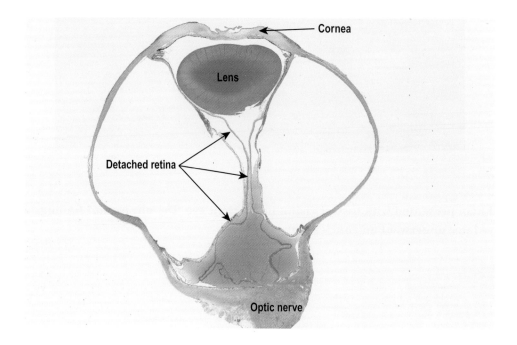

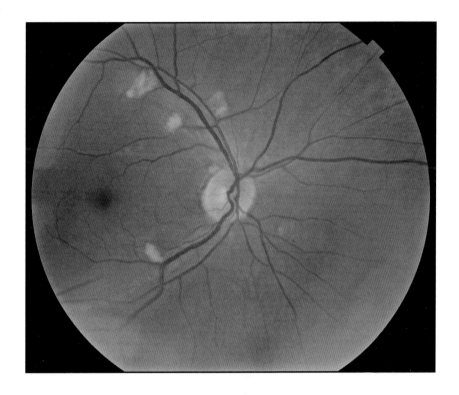

A 71-year-old man with a longstanding history of hypertension presented for a routine eye examination.

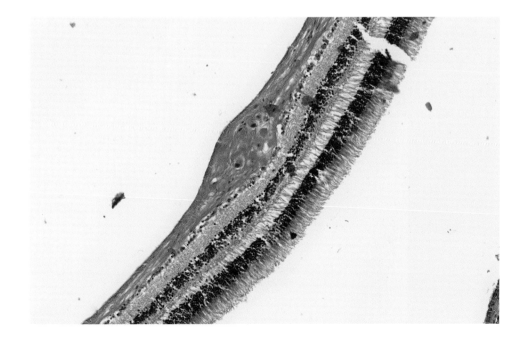

Diagnosis: Cotton-wool spots.

Clinical description: Fundus examination reveals multiple fluffy white patches.

Histological description: Cytoid bodies which are swelled axons are seen (circles). The cytoid bodies form as a result of nerve fiber layer ischemia and infarction.

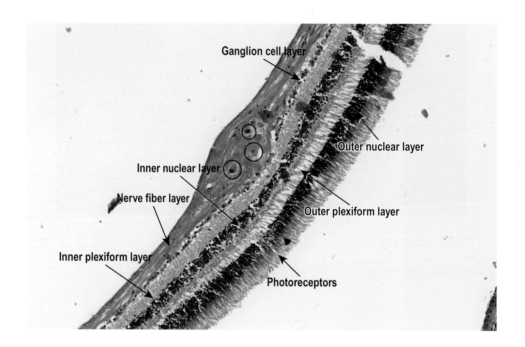

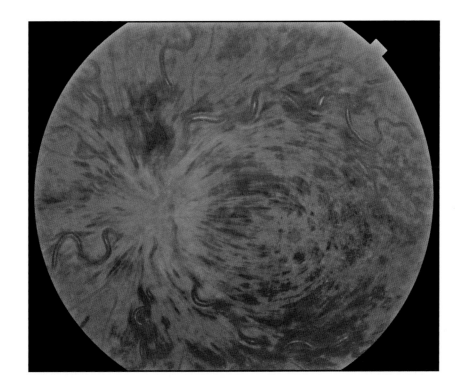

A 67-year-old man with a history of hypertension presented with decreased vision. Dilated fundus examination reveals the above findings.

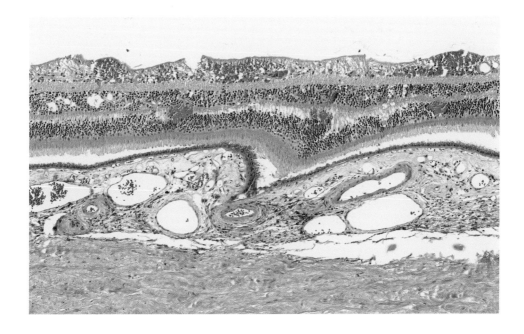

Diagnosis: Central retinal vein occlusion.

Clinical description: The fundus image demonstrates swelling of the optic nerve. Scattered hemorrhages in all retinal layers give it the classic "blood and thunder" appearance.

Histological description: Histopathology shows retinal hemorrhages in all retinal layers (asterisks).

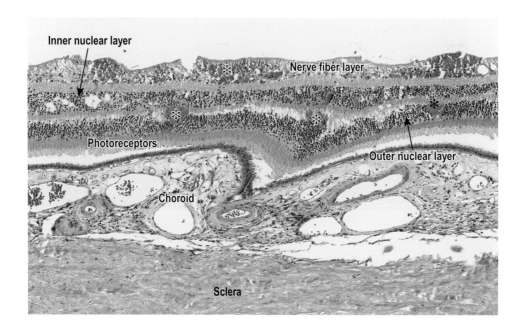

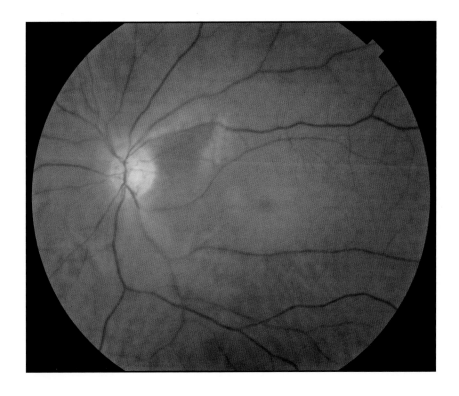

A 77-year-old woman presented with sudden loss of vision in her left eye and the fundus image shown above. Visual acuity was 20/20 OD and LP OS.

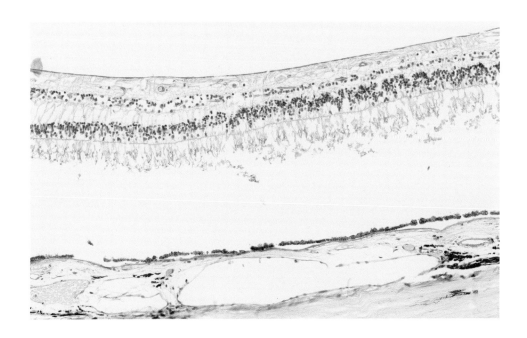

Diagnosis: Central retinal artery occlusion (CRAO).

Clinical description: The fundus examination demonstrates a cherry red spot typical for CRAO.

Histological description: Atrophy and ischemia of the inner retinal layers are most evident, although all layers are affected.

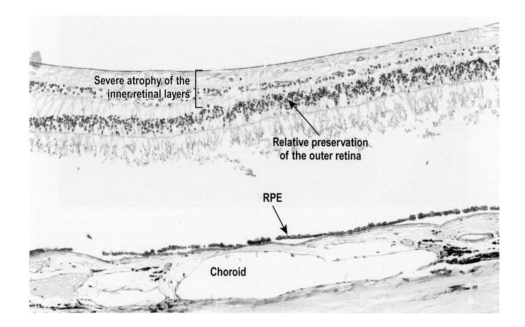

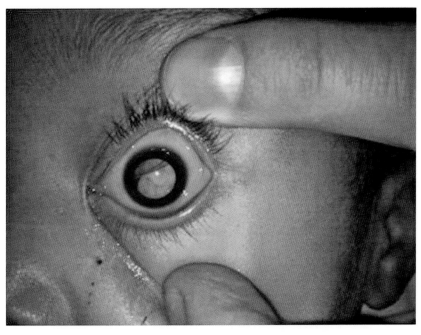

Courtesy of William R. Nunery, M.D. University of Louisville, Louisville KY.

A 2-year-old boy with a 6-month history of leukocoria was brought in by his mother.

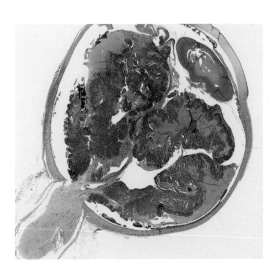 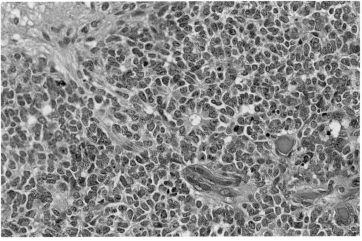

Diagnosis: Retinoblastoma.

Clinical description: Clinical examination demonstrates marked leukocoria.

Histological description: The slides reveal an enucleated globe with a large basophilic mass arising from the outer retina causing a complete retinal detachment and subretinal exudation (long arrow). Homer-Wright rosettes (short arrow), and Flexner-Wintersteiner rosettes (arrowhead) are seen.

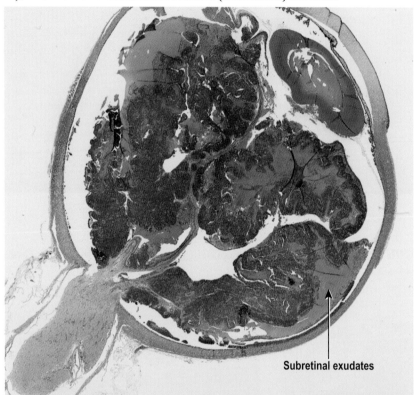

Subretinal exudates

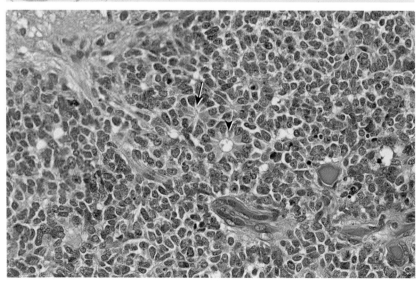

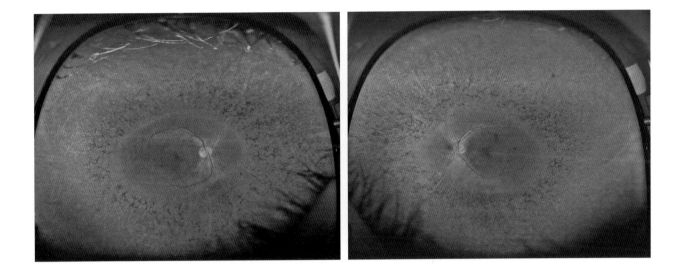

A 16-year-old boy presented with progressive loss of vision.

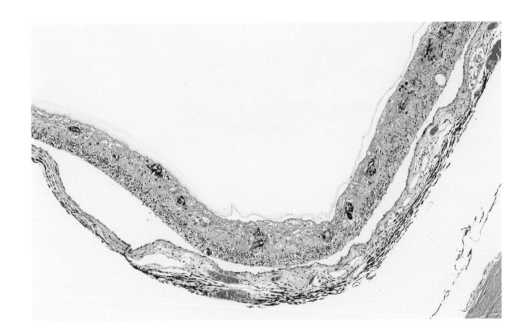

Diagnosis: Retinitis pigmentosa.

Clinical description: Fundus images reveal severely attenuated retinal vessel, waxy pallor of the optic disc, and "bone spicule" pigmentation in the periphery.

Histological description: There is severe and diffuse atrophy of the retinal photoreceptors, retinal pigmented epithelium, and outer nuclear layer. The retina is focally gliotic and there is a diffuse migration of the retinal pigmented epithelial cells around the hyalinized retinal vessels (arrowheads).

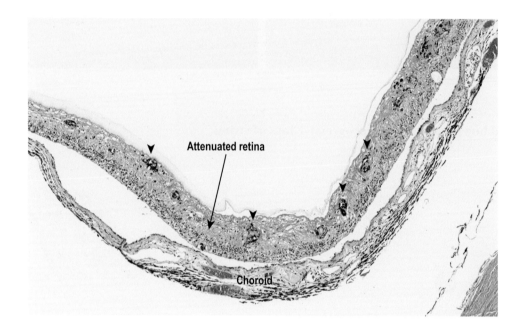

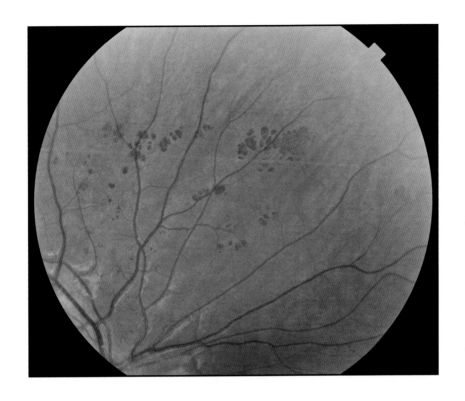

A 21-year-old woman presented with the above incidental retinal finding.

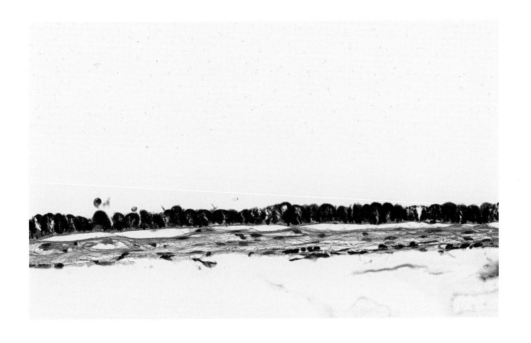

Diagnosis: Congenital hypertrophy of the retinal pigment epithelium (CHRPE).

Clinical description: Dilated fundus examination reveals multiple areas of grouped pigmented lesions giving a "bear track" appearance.

Histological description: Histopathology demonstrates hypertrophy and increased pigmentation of the retinal pigment epithelium.

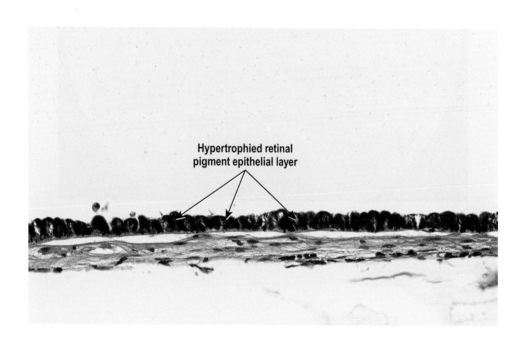

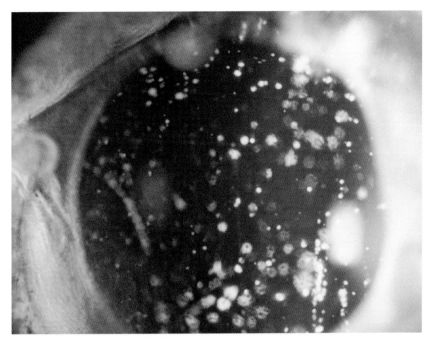

From Albert, Daniel M., Miller, Joan W., Azar, Dimitri T., and Blodi, Barbara A. (eds). 2008. Albert & Jakobiec's Principles and Practice of Ophthalmology, 3rd ed. Philadelphia: Copyright Elsevier 2008.

A 58-year-old man with no ocular complaints and normal visual acuity was seen for a routine eye examination. A slit-lamp image through his dilated pupil is shown.

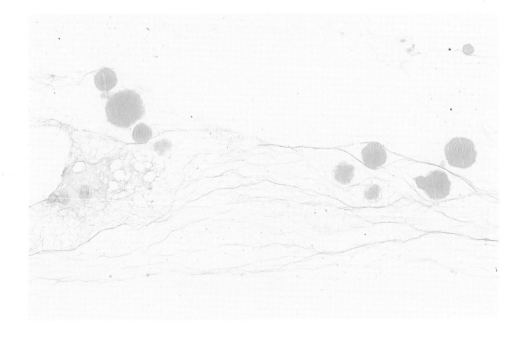

Diagnosis: Asteroid hyalosis.

Clinical description: The dilated slit-lamp examination reveals small round-to-oval asteroid bodies suspended in the vitreous.

Histological description: Histopathology demonstrates round, Alcian blue positive spheres (asterisks) consistent with asteroid bodies within the vitreous. Many of the asteroid bodies are attached to the vitreous.

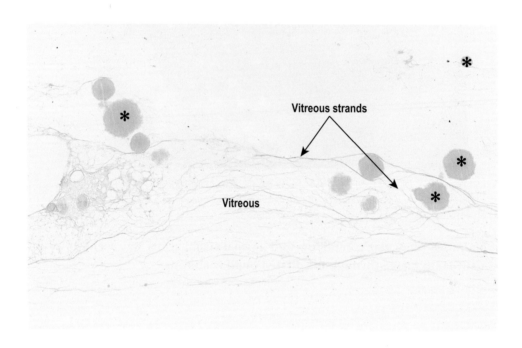

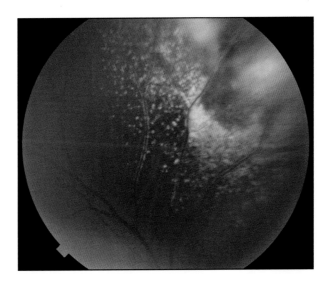

A 12-year-old boy presented with decreased vision and the above fundus finding.

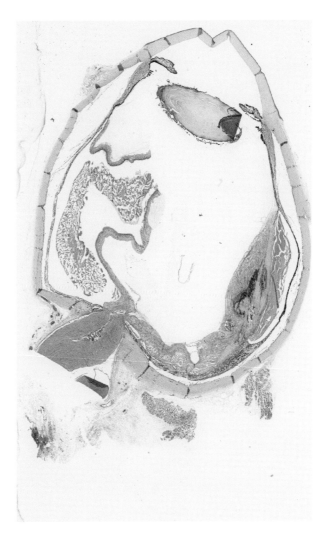

Diagnosis: Coats' disease.

Clinical description: Fundus image demonstrates retinal exudates.

Histological description: Histopathology demonstrates retinal detachment and subretinal exudates. Dilated telangiectatic blood vessels are also present.

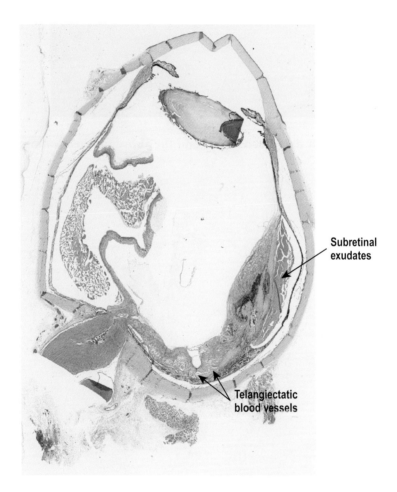

Subretinal exudates

Telangiectatic blood vessels

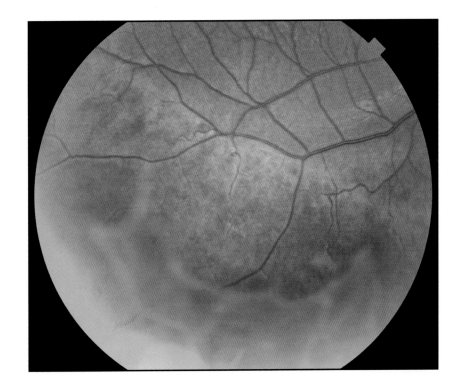

A 79-year-old man presented for a routine eye examination, with the above retinal finding.

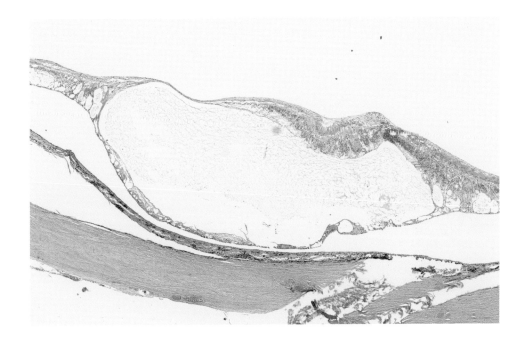

Diagnosis: Senile retinoschisis.

Clinical description: Fundus examination demonstrates smooth elevation of the retina inferiorly.

Histological description: Histopathology demonstrates splitting of the retina at the level of the outer plexiform layer (OPL).

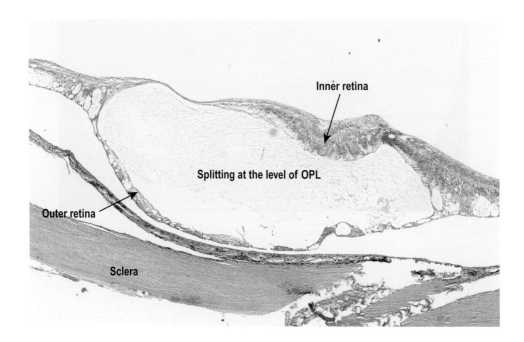

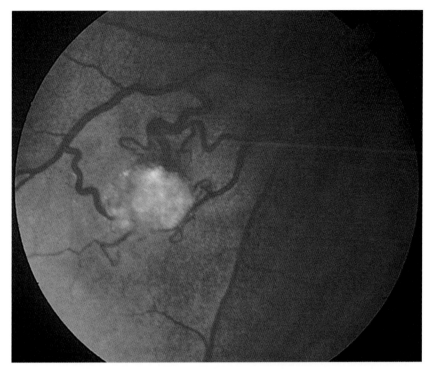

*From Albert, Daniel M., Miller, Joan W., Azar, Dimitri T., and Blodi, Barbara A. (eds). 2008. Albert
& Jakobiec's Principles and Practice of Ophthalmology, 3rd ed. Philadelphia: Copyright Elsevier 2008.*

A 33-year-old man presented with the above incidental finding on dilated fundus examination.

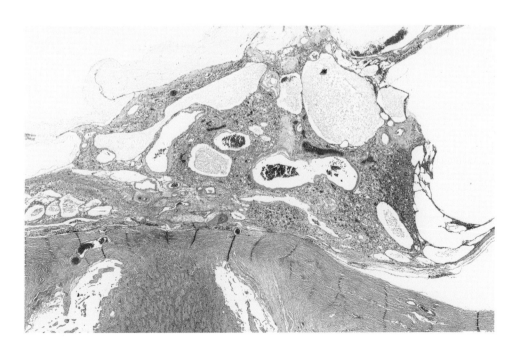

Diagnosis: Von Hippel–Lindau disease.

Clinical description: The fundus examination reveals dilated retinal vessels feeding a retinal hemangioblastoma in a patient with Von Hippel–Lindau disease.

Histological description: Histopathology demonstrates dilated vascular channels overlying the optic nerve (asterisks).

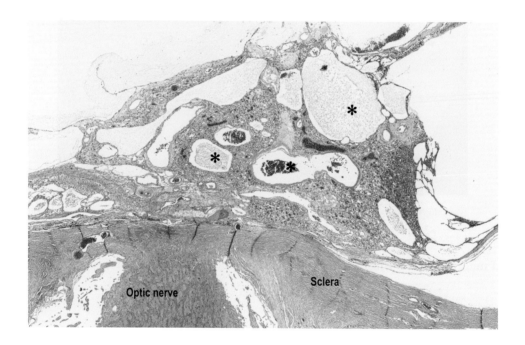

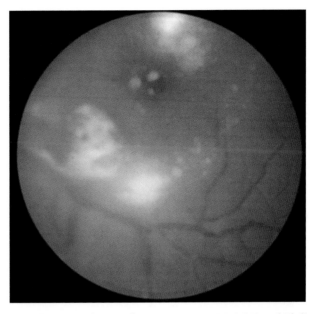

From Albert, Daniel M., Miller, Joan W., Azar, Dimitri T., and Blodi, Barbara A. (eds). 2008. Albert & Jakobiec's Principles and Practice of Ophthalmology, 3rd ed. Philadelphia: Copyright Elsevier 2008.

A 71-year-old renal transplant patient presented with decreased vision. Dilated fundus examination demonstrated the above findings.

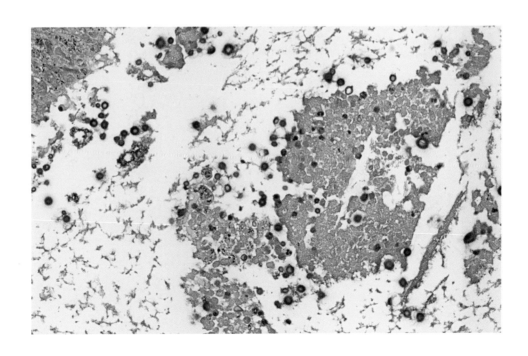

Diagnosis: Cryptococcal retinitis.

Clinical description: Dilated fundus examination demonstrates multifocal retinal infiltrates in this renal transplant patient.

Histological description: Histopathological examination demonstrates many well encapsulated cryptococcus organisms (arrows).

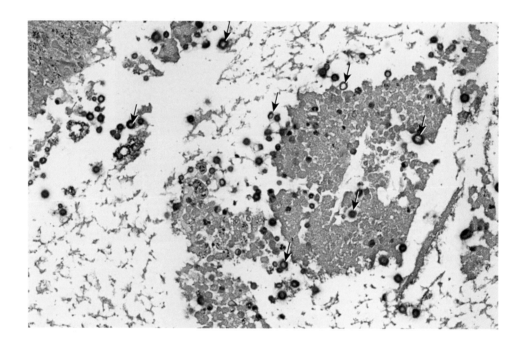

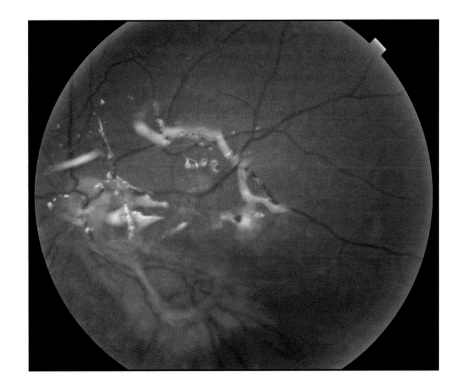

A 72-year-old woman presented with decreased vision and ocular pain. Doppler echocardiography was suspicious for endocarditis.

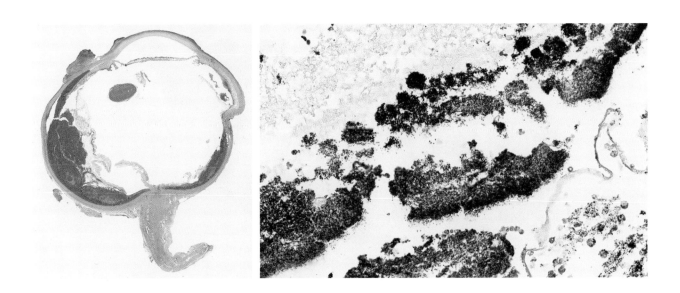

Diagnosis: Endogenous endophthalmitis.

Clinical description: Dilated fundus examination shows multiple cream-colored infiltrates within the vitreous.

Histological description: Histopathology demonstrates an enucleated eye with suprachoroidal hemorrhage, subretinal hemorrhage, and retinal detachment (top, asterisk). Gram stain demonstrates clusters of Gram-positive organisms within the vitreous (bottom).

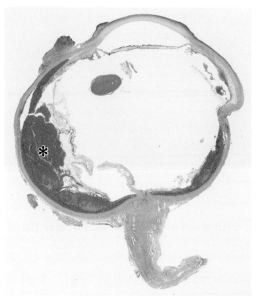

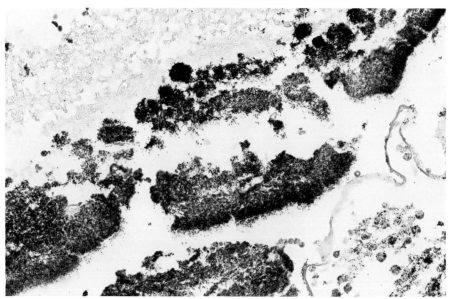

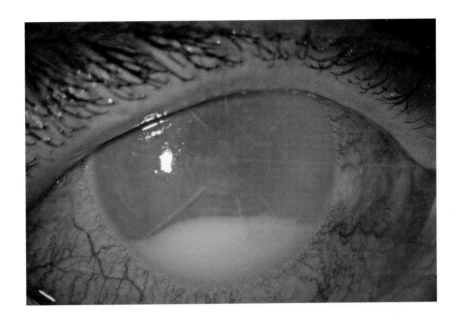

A 64-year-old patient presented with decreased vision and eye pain 3 days after a routine cataract surgery.

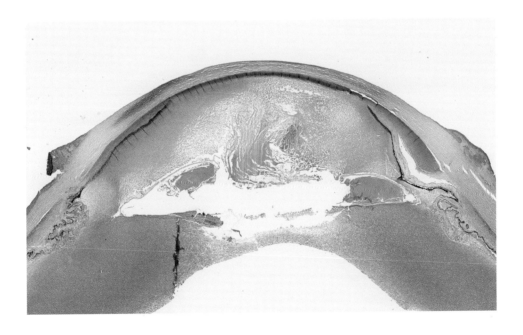

Diagnosis: Hypopyon with probable secondary endophthalmitis.

Clinical description: Slit-lamp examination reveals conjunctival hyperemia along with a hypopyon. Radial corneal scars consistent with previous radial keratotomy are seen.

Histological description: Histopathology demonstrates marked inflammation in the anterior chamber and the vitreous.

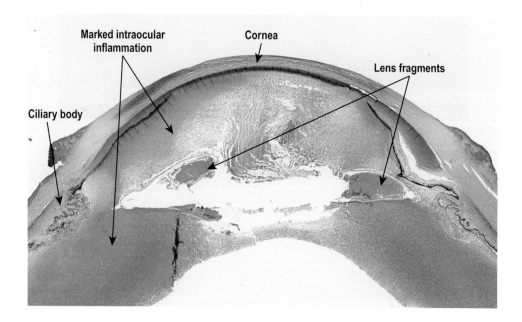

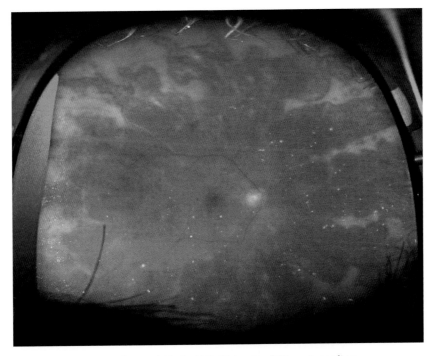

Courtesy of James A. Eadie, M.D. University of Wisconsin-Madison.

A 46-year-old man presented with a 1-week history of decreased vision, photophobia and ocular pain. On ophthalmic examination, he had variable amounts of vitritis in addition to the retinal findings shown above.

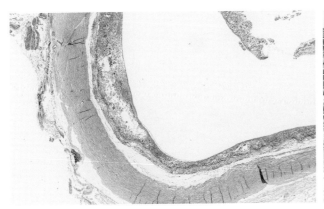

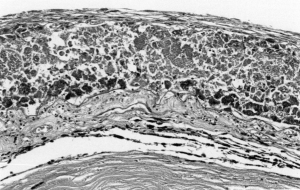

Diagnosis: Acute retinal necrosis (ARN).

Clinical description: Vitritis is seen, and the retina shows necrosis and opacification.

Histological description: Histopathology demonstrates necrosis and disorganization of all the retinal layers.

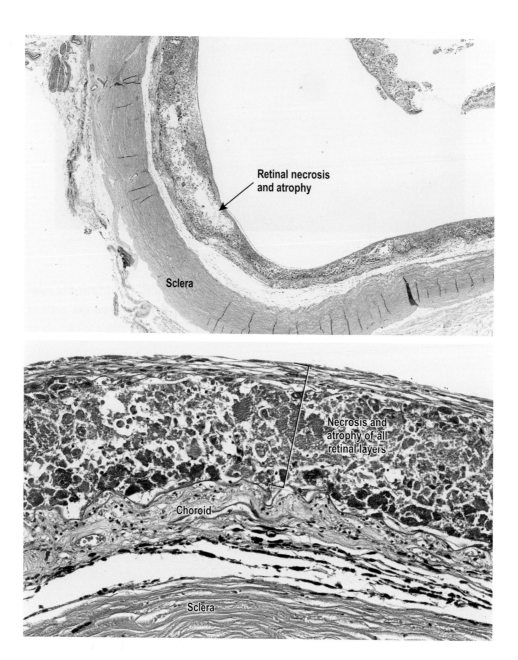

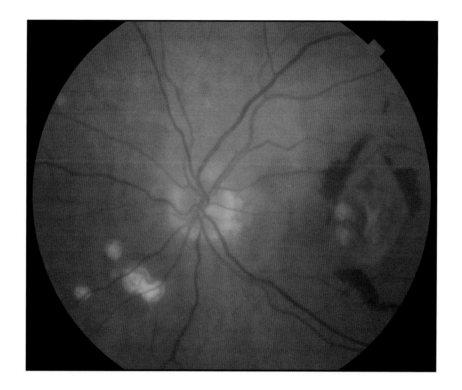

A 43-year-old woman from the Midwest United States presented with decreased vision.

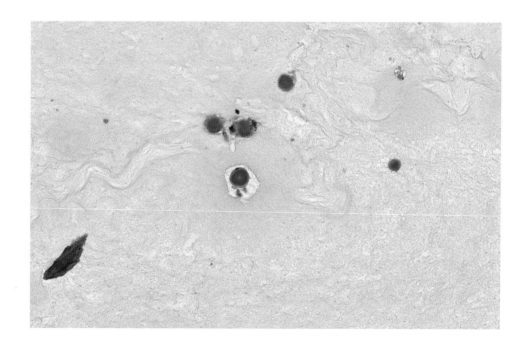

Diagnosis: Ocular histoplasmosis.

Clinical description: A dilated fundus examination reveals multiple punched out chorioretinal lesions in the periphery and within the macula. Hemorrhages and scarring are also present within the macular region.

Histological description: Histopathological evaluation reveals the *Histoplasma* capsulation organisms (arrows).

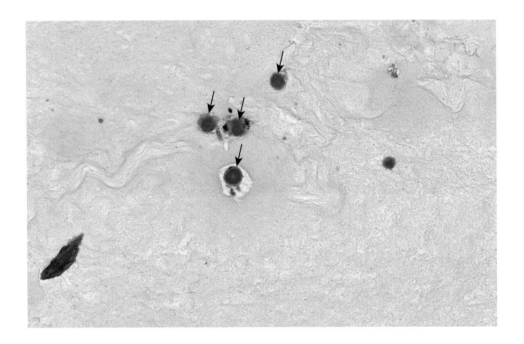

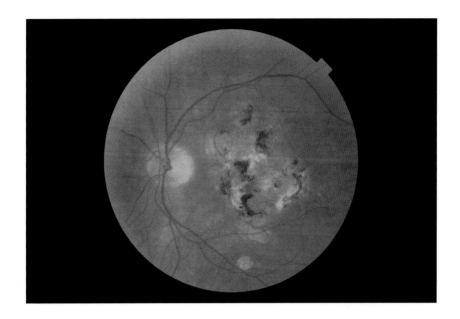

A 22-year-old man presented with a history of decreased vision in his left eye.

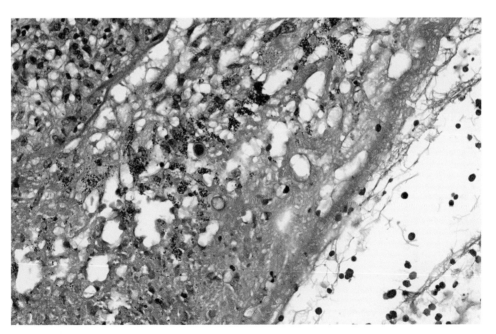

Courtesy of Mozhgan R. Kanavi, MD. Ophthalmic Research Center, Shahid Beheshti University of Medical Sciences, Tehran, Iran.

Diagnosis: Toxoplasma chorioretinitis.

Clinical description: Dilated fundus examination demonstrates extensive chorioretinal scarring in the macular region in this patient.

Histological description: Histopathology reveals disorganized retinal tissue with the presence of occasional toxoplasma cysts (arrows).

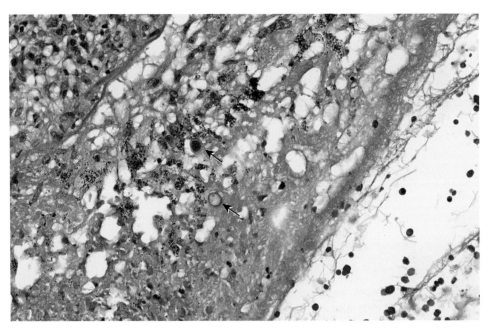

Courtesy of Mozhgan R. Kanavi, MD. Ophthalmic Research Center, Shahid Beheshti University of Medical Sciences, Tehran, Iran.

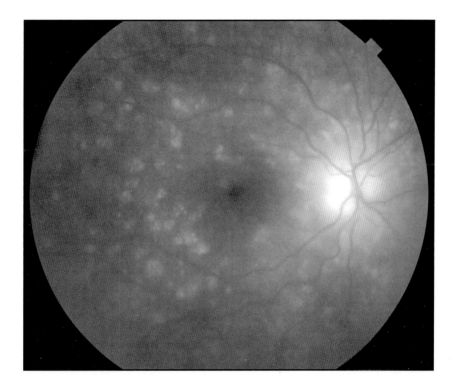

A 58-year-old patient presents with decreased vision, photophobia, and pain in his right eye. The patient had a history of a left ruptured globe 9 years ago. The fluorescein angiogram of the right eye is shown above.

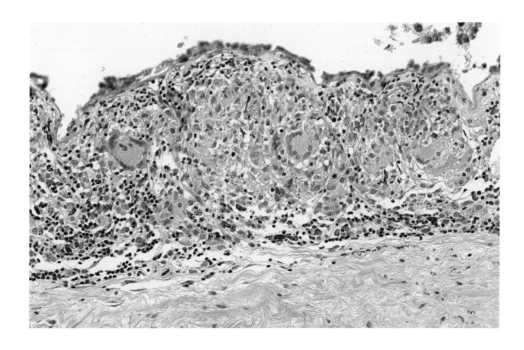

Diagnosis: Sympathetic ophthalmia.

Clinical description: Fluorescein angiogram demonstrates multiple areas of leakage consistent with serous retinal detachment.

Histological description: Histopathological examination reveals marked granulomatous inflammation, consisting of histiocytes and multinucleated giant cells, within the choroid. The choriocapillaris is relatively spared.

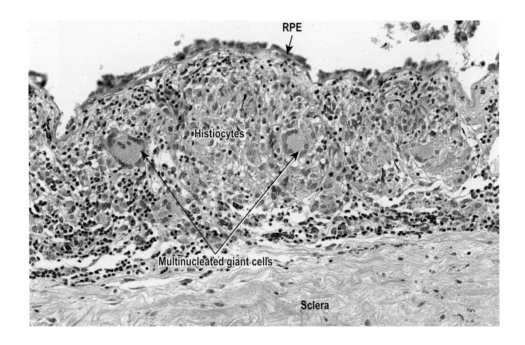

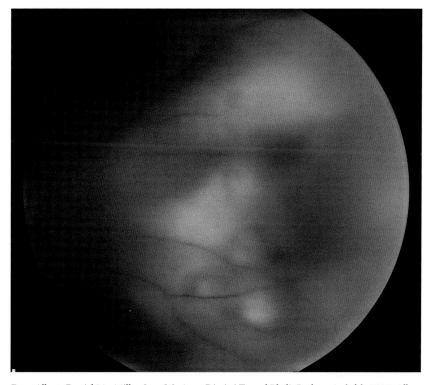

From Albert, Daniel M., Miller, Joan W., Azar, Dimitri T., and Blodi, Barbara A. (eds). 2008. Albert & Jakobiec's Principles and Practice of Ophthalmology, 3rd ed. Philadelphia: Copyright Elsevier 2008.

A 77-year-old patient with a history of chronic leukemia presented with decreased vision.

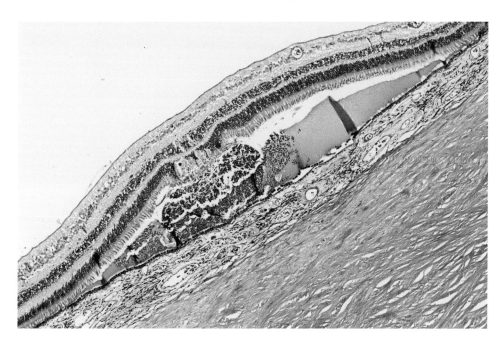

Diagnosis: Leukemia.

Clinical description: Dilated fundus examination reveals vitreous haze and multiple nodular choroidal infiltrates.

Histological description: Histopathology demonstrates exudative retinal detachment. Infiltration of the choroid and subretinal space with many leukemic cells is seen.

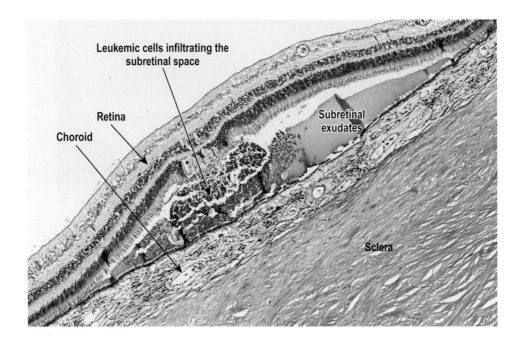

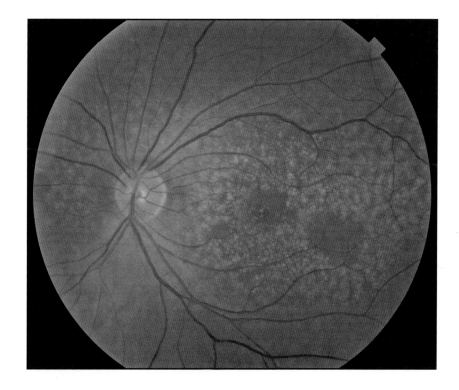

An 85-year-old woman presented for a routine eye examination. The appearance of the fundus is shown above. Fundus examination of her right eye revealed similar findings.

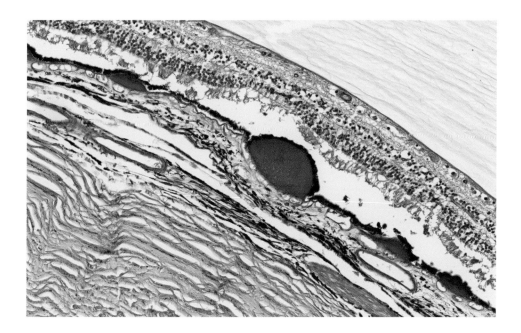

Diagnosis: Drusen.

Clinical description: The fundus examination reveals numerous yellow deposits within the macula consistent with drusen.

Histological description: Histopathology demonstrates multiple PAS-positive sub-RPE material consistent with drusen (asterisks).

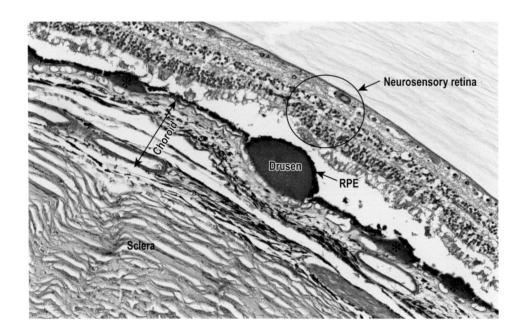

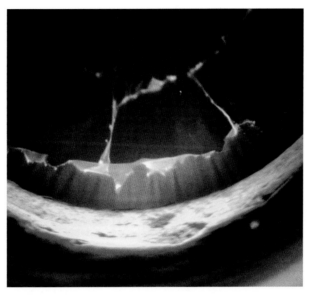

From Kanski JJ. Signs in Ophthalmology: Causes and Differential Diagnosis. Intraocular Pressure and Angle. Philadelphia: Copyright Elsevier 2010.

An elderly woman presented with elevated IOP and the above slit-lamp appearance.

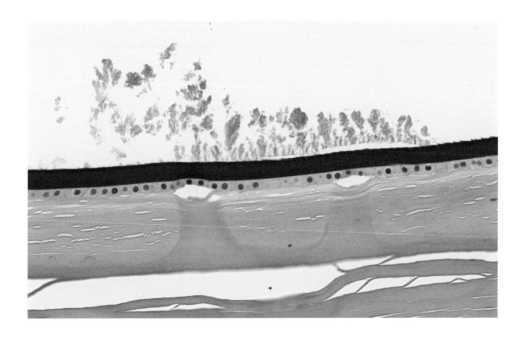

Diagnosis: Pseudoexfoliation syndrome.

Clinical description: The slit-lamp examination demonstrates the presence of pseudoexfoliative material on the anterior lens capsule.

Histological description: Histopathology demonstrates deposition of amorphous pseudoexfoliative material on the anterior lens capsule resembling iron filings aligned on a magnet (arrows).

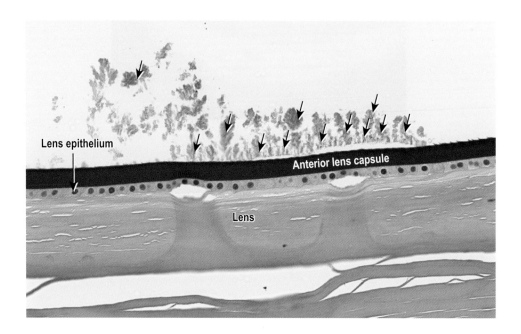

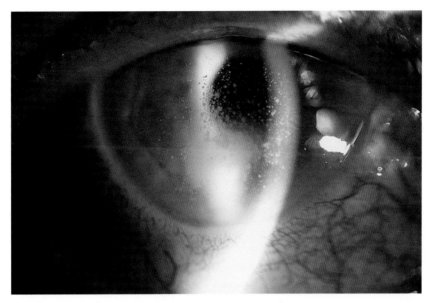

From Albert, Daniel M., Miller, Joan W., Azar, Dimitri T., and Blodi, Barbara A. (eds). 2008. Albert & Jakobiec's Principles and Practice of Ophthalmology, 3rd ed. Philadelphia: Copyright Elsevier 2008.

A 68-year-old woman presented with decreased vision, photophobia, and eye pain after a complicated cataract surgery.

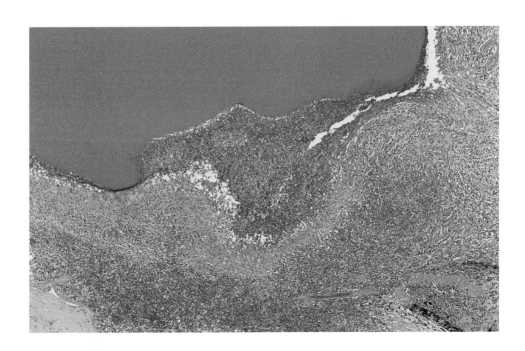

Diagnosis: Phacoantigenic uveitis.

Clinical description: Slit-lamp examination demonstrates corneal edema with presence of many keratic precipitates and anterior chamber haze.

Histological description: Histopathology demonstrates zonular pattern of granulomatous inflammation, composed of neutrophils, lymphocytes, and plasma cells as well as epithelioid cells surrounding the lens. Remnants of broken lens capsule are also seen.

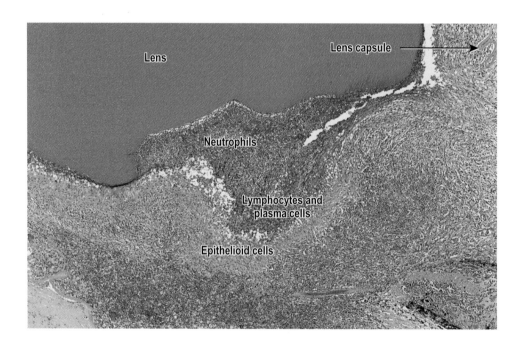

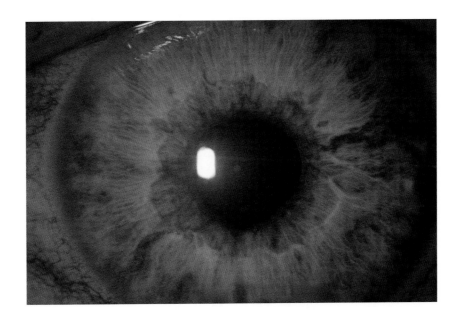

A 58-year-old man with a past medical history of hypertension and insulin-dependent diabetes mellitus presented with decreased vision and eye pain. IOP was measured to be 65 mmHg.

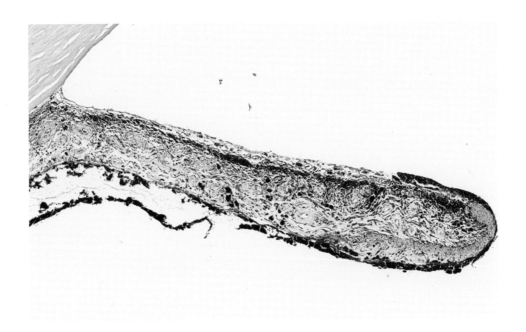

Diagnosis: Neovascular glaucoma.

Clinical description: Clinical examination demonstrates florid iris rubeosis.

Histological description: Histopathology reveals an iris tissue with ectropion uveae. Marked iris neovascularization (arrowheads) and peripheral anterior synechiae closing the angle are present.

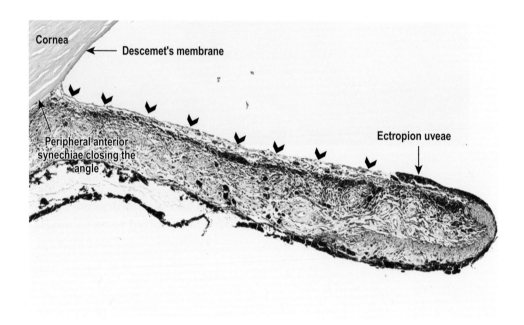

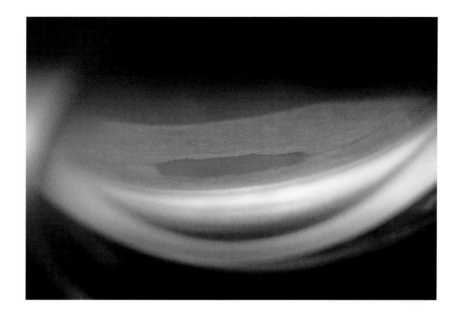

A 16-year-old patient presented with the above gonioscopic findings following a blunt eye trauma.

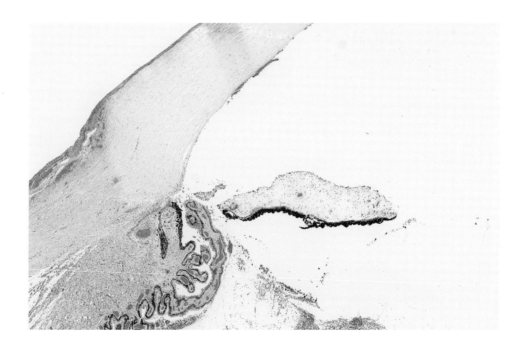

Diagnosis: Iridodialysis.

Clinical description: Gonioscopic examination reveals separation of the iris from its base.

Histological description: Histopathology demonstrates a detached iris.

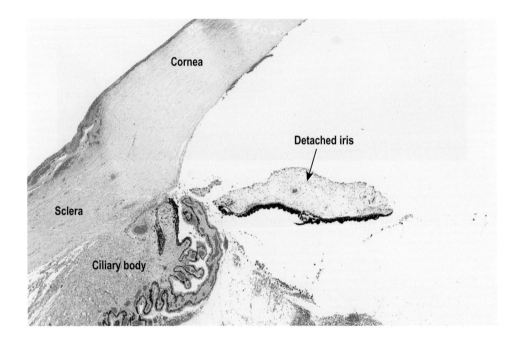

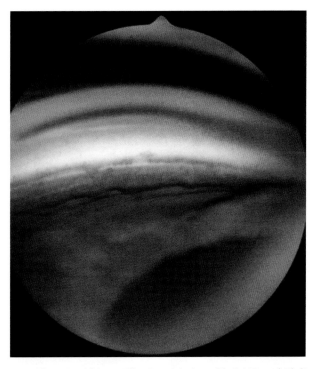

From Albert, Daniel M., Miller, Joan W., Azar, Dimitri T., and Blodi,
Barbara A. (eds). 2008. Albert & Jakobiec's Principles and Practice of
Ophthalmology, 3rd ed. Philadelphia: Copyright Elsevier 2008.

A 19-year-old patient presented to his ophthalmologist following a blunt ocular trauma.

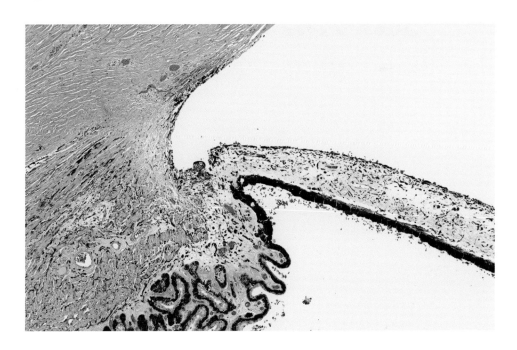

Diagnosis: Angle recession.

Clinical description: Gonioscopic examination reveals widening of the ciliary body band consistent with angle recession.

Histological description: Histopathology demonstrates a tear into the face of the ciliary body resulting in a cleavage between circular and longitudinal ciliary body muscles (arrow).

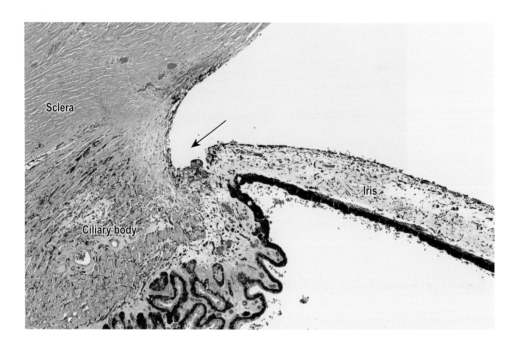

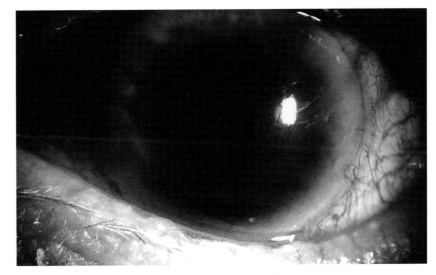

Courtesy of Neal P. Barney, M.D. University of Wisconsin-Madison.

A 56-year-old man sustained an ocular injury. He later developed an elevated IOP and ocular pain.

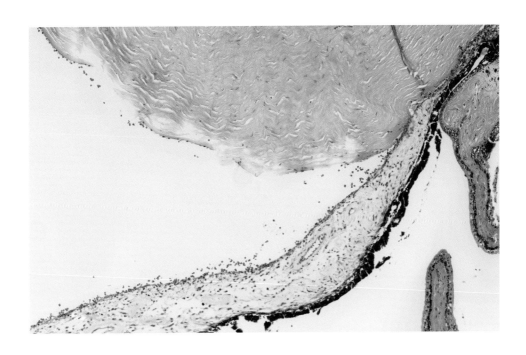

Diagnosis: Hemorrhagic glaucoma.

Clinical description: Slit-lamp examination demonstrates hyphema with layering of the blood in the anterior chamber.

Histological description: Histopathological evaluation shows blood in the anterior chamber and within the angle (arrows).

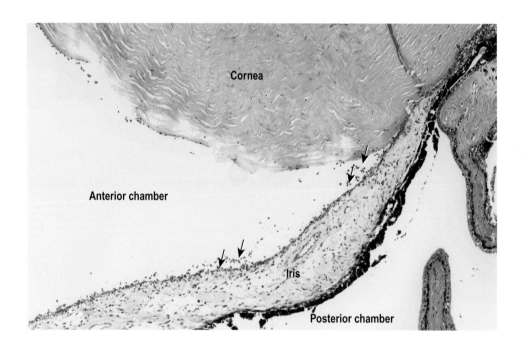

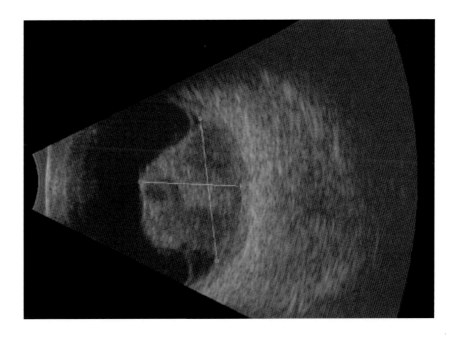

A 55-year-old man presented with decreased vision and ocular pain. An intraocular mass was discovered on examination.

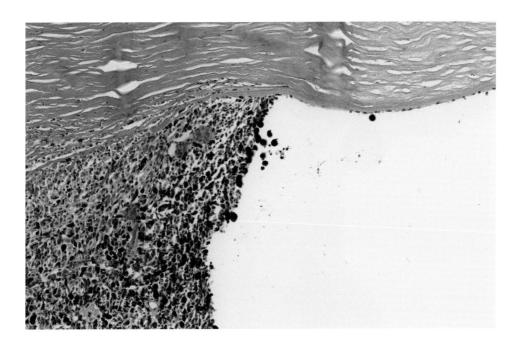

Diagnosis: Melanocytic glaucoma.

Clinical description: Ultrasound reveals a large choroidal lesion most consistent with choroidal melanoma.

Histological description: Histopathology demonstrates numerous pigment-laden macrophages within the trabecular meshwork and the anterior chamber.

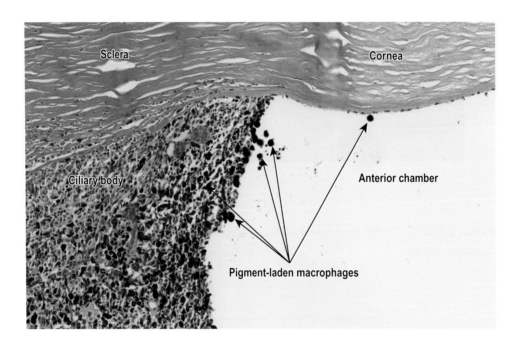

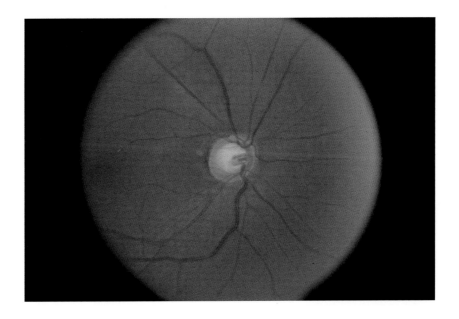

The patient is a 72-year-old man with gradual loss of vision despite maximum medical and surgical therapy.

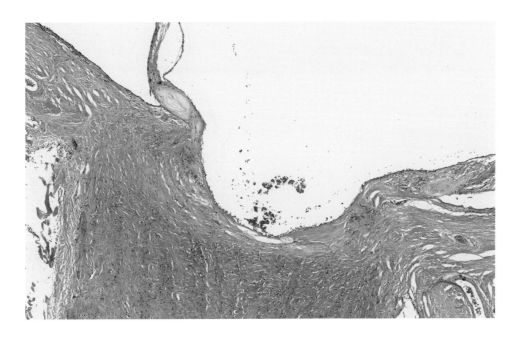

Diagnosis: Optic disc cupping secondary to glaucoma.

Clinical description: The optic nerve head is severely cupped with only a small rim of normal tissue remaining.

Histological description: An excavated optic nerve head is evident on this histopathologic section (arrows) as well as atrophy of the optic nerve.

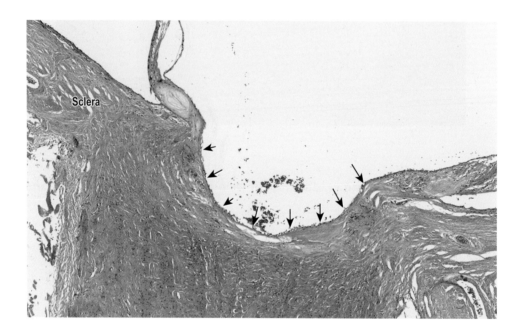

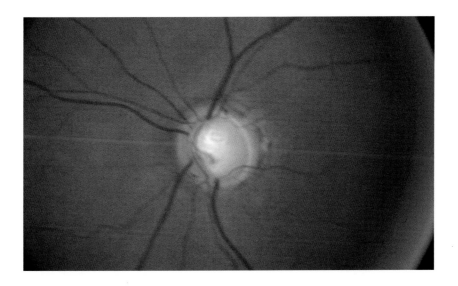

A 77-year-old man with a history of angle closure glaucoma presented with decreased vision and restricted visual fields. A few years later he underwent enucleation.

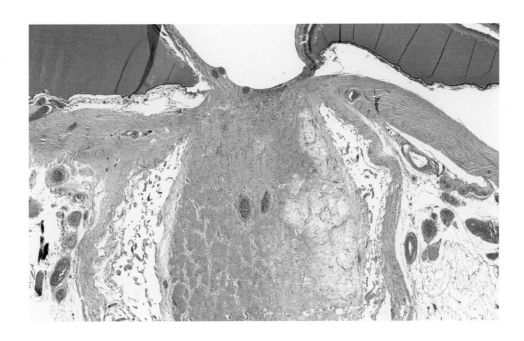

Diagnosis: Schnabel's cavernous dystrophy.

Clinical description: Dilated fundus examination shows a pale optic nerve with severe excavation and cupping.

Histological description: Histopathology reveals Schnabel's cavernous degeneration of the retrolaminar optic nerve exhibiting spongiform changes (asterisks).

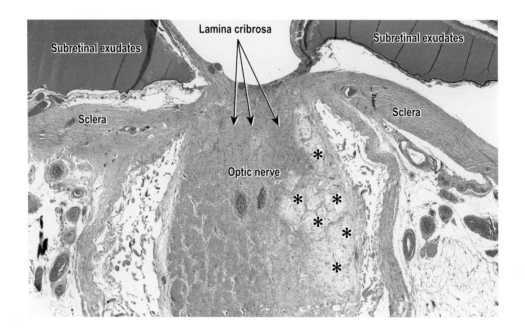

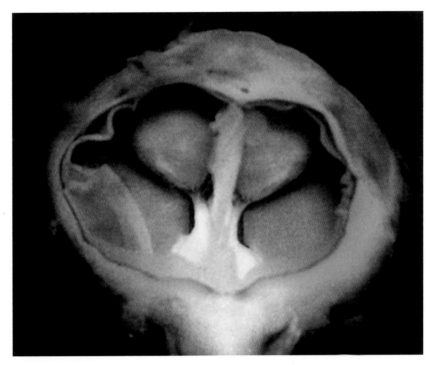

From Albert, Daniel M., Miller, Joan W., Azar, Dimitri T., and Blodi, Barbara A. (eds). 2008. Albert & Jakobiec's Principles and Practice of Ophthalmology, 3rd ed. Philadelphia: Copyright Elsevier 2008.

The above eye was removed from a stillborn fetus with multiple abnormalities.

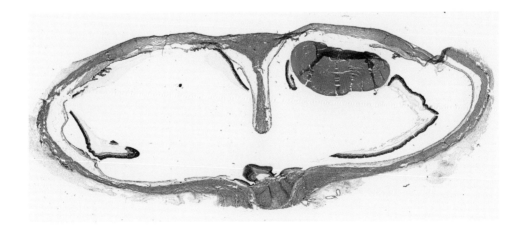

Diagnosis: Synophthalmos (Cyclopia).

Clinical description: The enucleated specimen shows fused globes.

Histological description: Histopathology demonstrates globes fused medially (asterisks) sharing a common optic nerve.

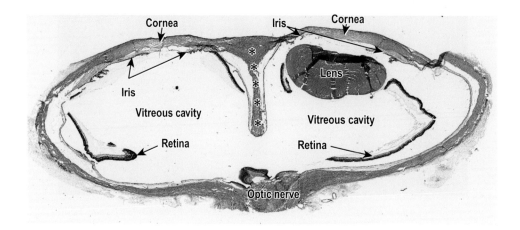

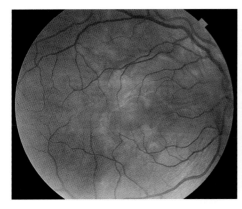

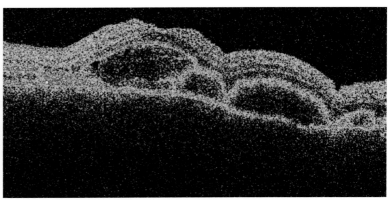

From Albert, Daniel M., Miller, Joan W., Azar, Dimitri T., and Blodi, Barbara A. (eds). 2008. Albert & Jakobiec's Principles and Practice of Ophthalmology, 3rd ed. Philadelphia: Copyright Elsevier 2008.

From Albert, Daniel M., Miller, Joan W., Azar, Dimitri T., and Blodi, Barbara A. (eds). 2008. Albert & Jakobiec's Principles and Practice of Ophthalmology, 3rd ed. Philadelphia: Copyright Elsevier 2008.

A 36-year-old patient with a history of chronic headache presented with decreased vision.

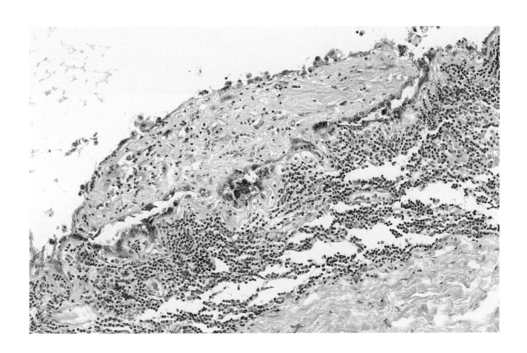

Diagnosis: Vogt–Koyanagi–Harada (VKH) syndrome.

Clinical description: Dilated fundus examination and OCT show multiple serous retinal detachments.

Histological description: Histopathology reveals collection of epithelioid cells under the RPE. The choroidal tissue is infiltrated with lymphoplasmacytic inflammation. Retinal inflammation is also present but not shown.

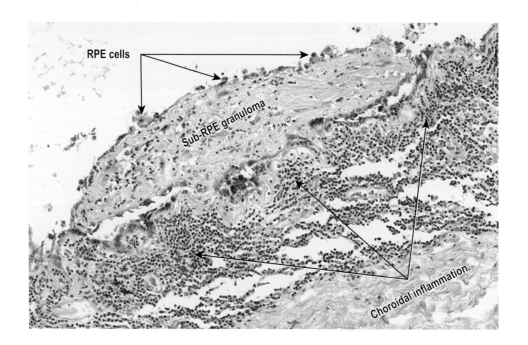

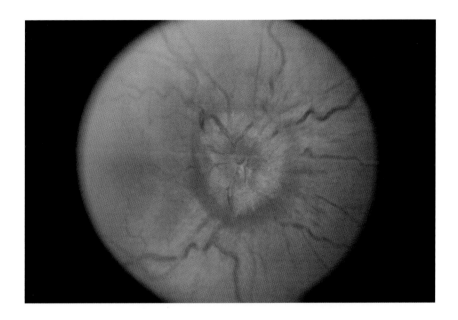

A 75-year-old woman presented with sudden loss of vision and a right afferent pupillary defect.

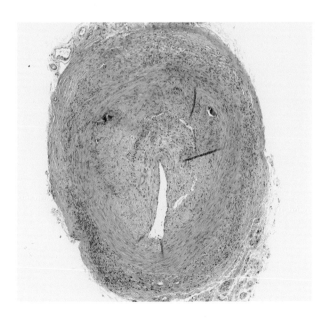

Diagnosis: Temporal (giant cell) arteritis.

Clinical description: The fundus examination reveals optic nerve edema.

Histological description: The temporal artery demonstrates thickening of intima, discontinuity in internal elastic lamina and granulomatous inflammation within the intima and media. Multinucleated giant cells are also seen.

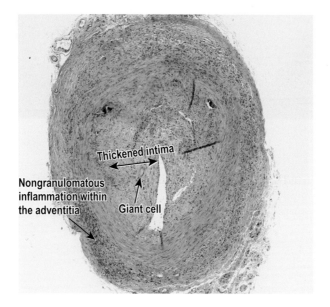

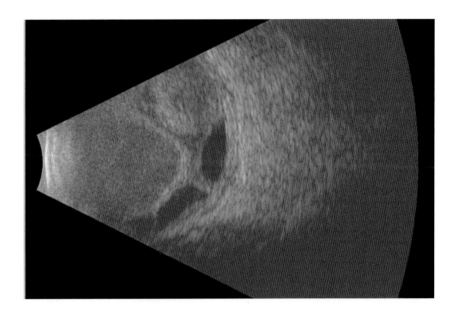

A 79-year-old woman presented with hypotony with the above ultrasound finding after a complicated cataract surgery.

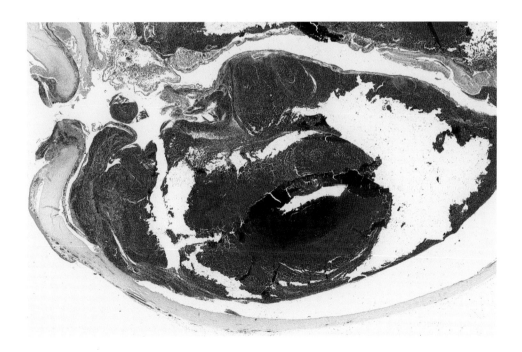

Diagnosis: Suprachoroidal hemorrhage.

Clinical description: Ultrasound demonstrates blood in the suprachoroidal space.

Histological description: Large amounts of hemorrhage are seen in the suprachoroidal space. Total retinal detachment is present.

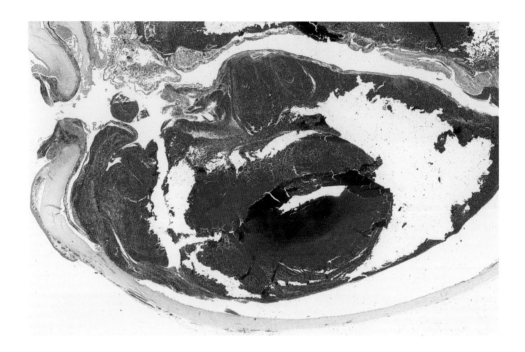

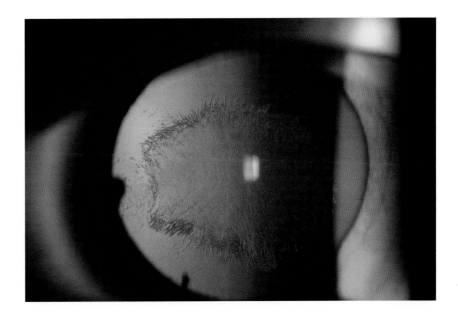

A 67-year-old woman presented with decreased vision and difficulty driving at night. A slit-lamp view of the lens is shown above.

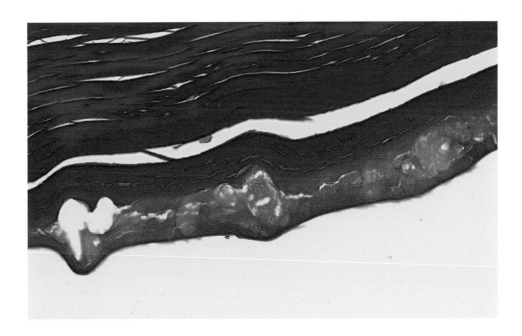

Diagnosis: Posterior subcapsular cataract.

Clinical description: Dilated slit-lamp examination demonstrates a posterior subcapsular opacity.

Histological description: Histopathology shows collection of morgagnian globules (asterisks) in the posterior aspect of the lens (arrow).

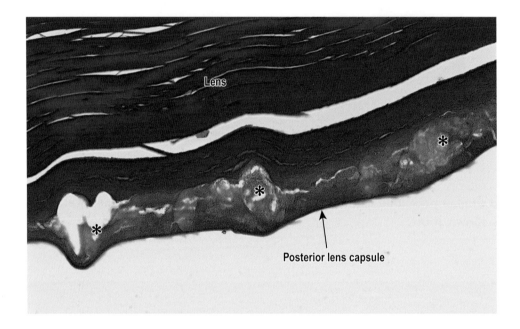

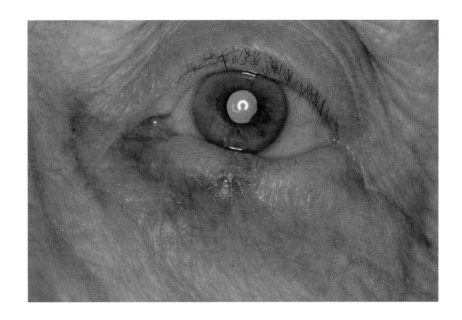

An 87-year-old man presented with difficulty seeing at both distance and near.

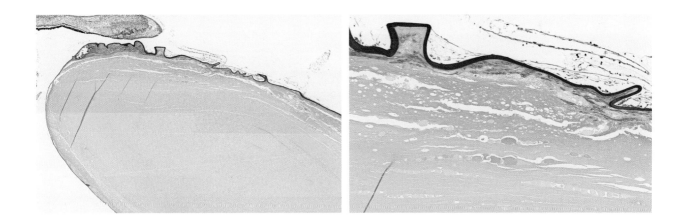

Diagnosis: Hypermature cataract.

Clinical description: Slit-lamp examination shows a white mature cataract in this patient.

Histological description: Histological examination reveals an enlarged lens with morgagnian globules (asterisks) consistent with cataract.

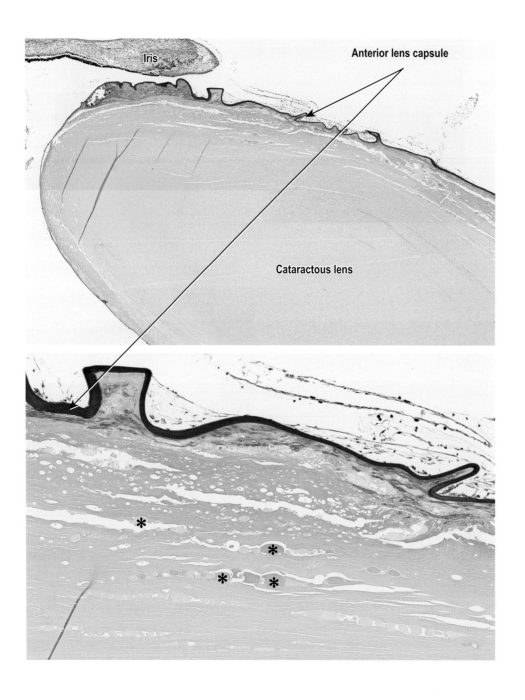

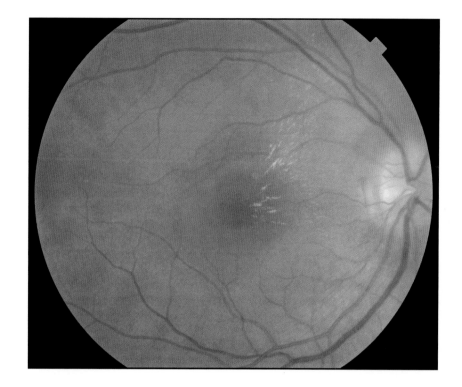

A 55-year-old man with a history of chronic diarrhea presented with decreased vision for the past 4 months.

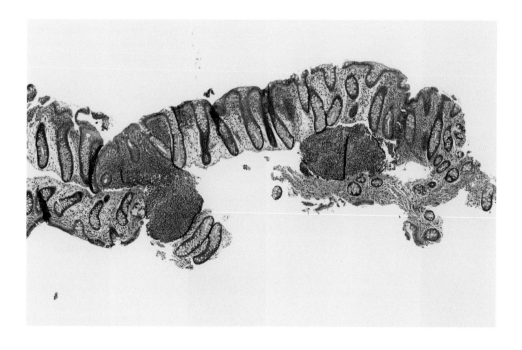

Diagnosis: Crohn's disease.

Clinical description: Exudates forming a macular star are seen on the dilated fundus examination.

Histological description: Intestinal biopsy reveals inflammation within the lamina propria. Peyer's patches, which are a normal finding, are also seen.

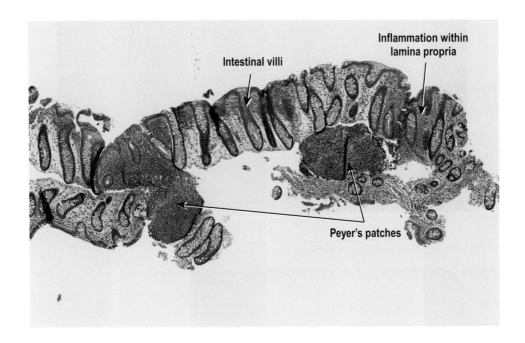

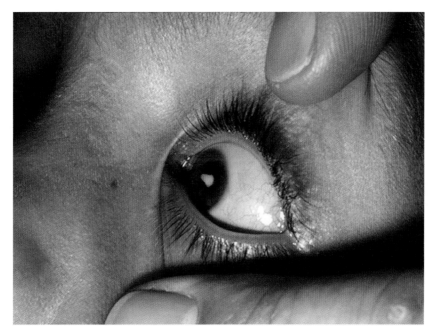

From Albert, Daniel M., Miller, Joan W., Azar, Dimitri T., and Blodi, Barbara A. (eds). 2008. Albert & Jakobiec's Principles and Practice of Ophthalmology, 3rd ed. Philadelphia: Copyright Elsevier 2008.

An 8-year-old patient presented with decreased vision and amblyopia.

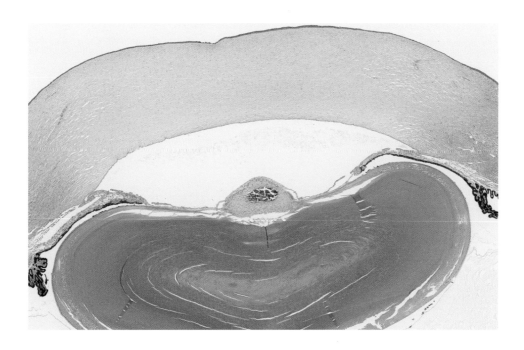

Diagnosis: Anterior polar cataract.

Clinical description: Slit-lamp examination reveals an anteriorly located lens opacity in the pupillary space.

Histological description: Histopathology reveals calcification and cellular proliferation under the anterior lens capsule.

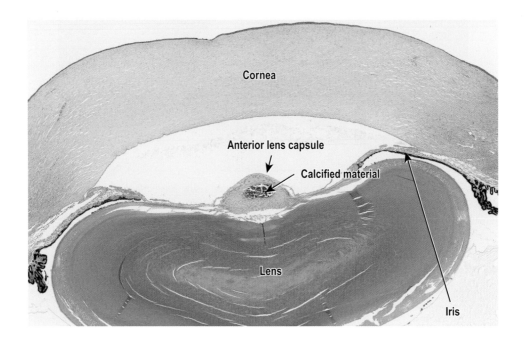

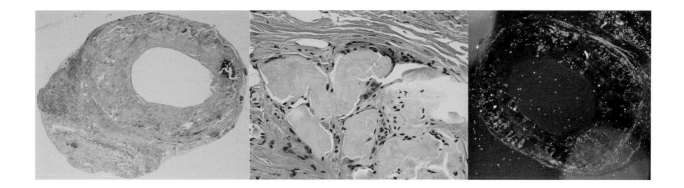

A 66-year-old man with a history of multiple myeloma presented with decreased vision, headaches, and jaw claudication.

Diagnosis: Amyloid deposits in the temporal artery.

Clinical description: The fundus image shows optic nerve edema with a small peripapillary hemorrhage and a supratemporal cotton-wool spot. The visual field is significant for a complete superior altitudinal defect.

Histological description: Histopathology demonstrates infiltration of amorphous material within the tunica intima, tunica media, and tunica adventitia (left). Higher magnification shows giant cells surrounding the amorphous eosinophilic deposits (center). Amyloid staining with Congo red produces birefringence under polarized light (right).

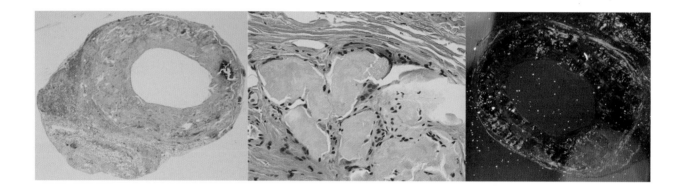

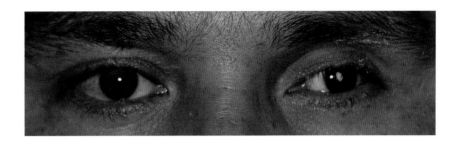

A 28-year-old man presented with a blind painful left eye.

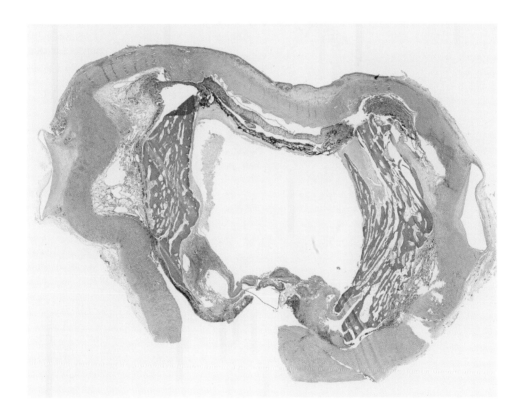

Diagnosis: Phthisis bulbi.

Clinical description: Clinical examination reveals left enophthalmos and exotropia in this patient.

Histological description: Histopathological examination reveals marked osseous RPE metaplasia producing a cancellous bone shell in the vitreous cavity. The retina is detached, disorganized, and atrophic. The sclera is thickened and folded and a mild chronic lymphocytic infiltrate is present.

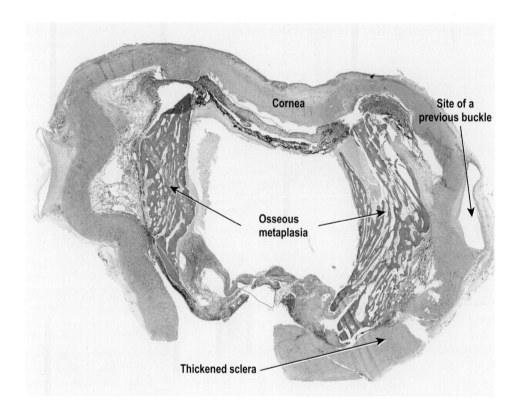

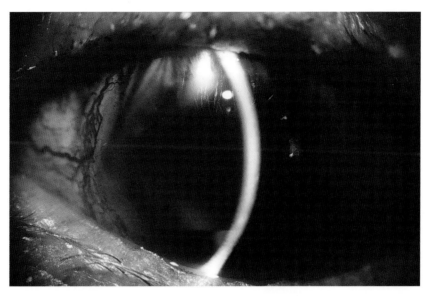

Courtesy of Neal P. Barney, M.D. University of Wisconsin-Madison.

A 22-year-old man presented with pain and decreased vision after blunt trauma to his eye.

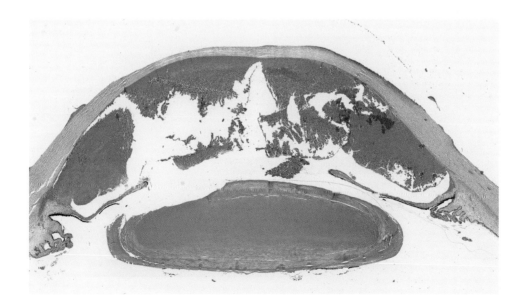

Diagnosis: Hyphema.

Clinical description: Layering of blood is noted within the anterior chamber.

Histological description: Histopathology demonstrates marked hemorrhage in the anterior chamber.

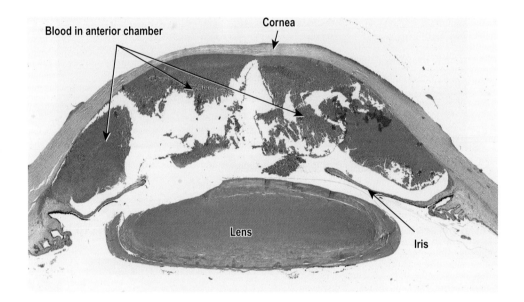

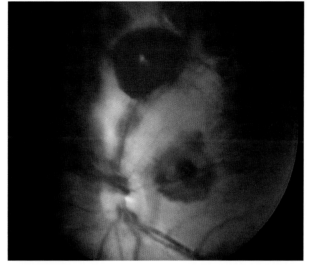

From Albert, Daniel M., Miller, Joan W., Azar, Dimitri T., and Blodi, Barbara A. (eds). 2008. Albert & Jakobiec's Principles and Practice of Ophthalmology, 3rd ed. Philadelphia: Copyright Elsevier 2008.

An unconscious 4-month-old infant was brought to ER by her caregiver.

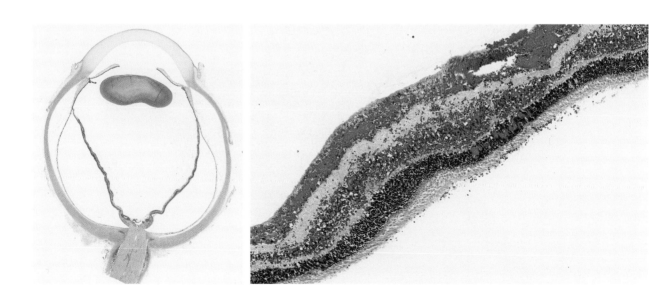

Diagnosis: Abusive head trauma (a.k.a shaken baby syndrome).

Clinical description: Dilated fundus examination reveals massive retinal hemorrhages affecting all layers.

Histological description: Histopathology reveals hemorrhages affecting all retinal layers and the optic nerve sheath. The retinal hemorrhages extend to the ora serrata (asterisks).

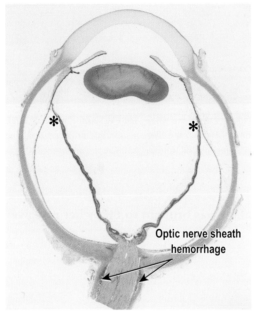

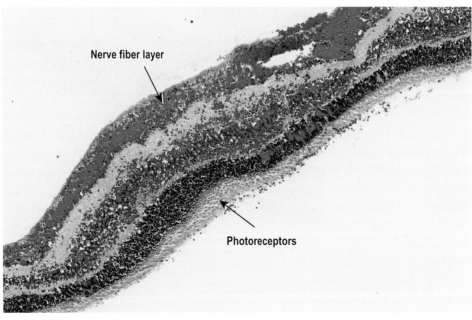

Index of cases

Index

Page numbers followed by "f" indicate figures.

A

Abusive head trauma, 399f–400f, 400
Acanthamoeba keratitis, 173f–174f, 174
Acanthosis, 4, 16f, 18, 22f, 24f, 52f, 238f, 270f
Acanthotic epithelium, 240, 240f
Acanthotic lobules, of epithelial cells, 56f
Acanthotic skin epithelium, 6f
Acquired immunodeficiency syndrome (AIDS), 179, 179f
Actinic keratosis, 3f–4f, 4
Actinomyces, canaliculitis secondary to, 113f, 114
Acute nongranulomatous inflammation, 260
Acute retinal necrosis, 347f–348f, 348
Adenoid cystic carcinoma, 87f–88f, 88
Adenoma, pleomorphic, 83f–84f, 84
Adipose tissue, lobules of, 94, 94f
Afferent pupillary defect, 381
Alcian blue staining, 142
ALHE. *see* Angiolymphoid hyperplasia with eosinophilia (ALHE).
Amblyopia, 391
Amorphous eosinophilic substance, 266f
Amyloid deposits, in temporal artery, 393f–394f, 394
Amyloidosis, conjunctival, 233f–234f, 234
Angiolymphoid hyperplasia with eosinophilia (ALHE), 81f–82f, 82
Angle closure glaucoma, 375
Angle recession, 367f–368f, 368
Anterior basement membrane dystrophy, 143f–144f, 144
Anterior chamber, 370f, 372f
    blood in, 398f
Anterior corneal nodules, 150
Anterior lens capsule, 360f, 388f, 392f
Anterior orbitotomy, with left upper eyelid fullness, 111, 111f
Anterior polar cataract, 391f–392f, 392
Anterior stromal opacities, 138
Apical snouts, 38f
Apocrine hidrocystoma, 37f–38f, 38
Aspergillus, fungal keratitis secondary to, 176

Asteroid bodies, attached to vitreous, 334, 334f
Asteroid hyalosis, 333f–334f, 334
Astigmatism, irregular, 201, 201f
Atypical basaloid cells, 32
Avellino corneal dystrophy, 139f–140f, 140

B

Bacterial conjunctivitis, 261f–262f, 262
Bacterial keratitis, 181f–182f, 182
Balloon cell melanoma, 305f–306f, 306
Band keratopathy, 145f–146f, 146
Basal cell carcinoma, 1f–2f, 2
    morpheaform, 27f–28f, 28
    pigmented, 31f–32f, 32
Basal epithelial pigmentation, 20f
Basaloid cells
    in adenoid cystic carcinoma, 88f
    foamy cells lined by, 30f
    islands of, 2f
    with peripheral palisading of nuclei, 48f
Basophilic cells, 46f
"Beaten bronze" appearance, 160
Benign acquired melanosis (BAM), 213f–214f, 214
Benign mixed tumor. *see* Pleomorphic adenoma.
Benign reactive lymphoid hyperplasia (BRLH), 251f–252f, 252
Bilateral diffuse uveal melanocytic proliferation (BDUMP), 283f–284f, 284
Biopsy
    excisional, with left upper eyelid fullness, 83
    orbital
        histiocytic cell tumor in, 110
        with increasing proptosis, 91, 91f
Blood, in anterior chamber, 398f
Blood vessel lumen, 76f
Blood vessels
    dilated thick-walled, in cavernous hemangioma of the orbit, 92
    radiating, 260, 260f
Bowman's layer, 144f, 146, 180f
    loss of, 158
Bowman's membrane, 150

Breast cancer, 311
    metastatic, to choroid, 311f–312f, 312
    with orbital cancer, 123f–124f, 124
Burkitt's lymphoma, 249f–250f, 250

C

Calcification, in pilomatrixoma, 46f
Calcified material, 392f
Calcified mineralized tissue, Gram-positive filaments in, 114, 114f
Canaliculitis secondary to *Actinomyces*, 113f, 114
Capillary hemangioma, of eyelid, 73f–74f, 74
Cardiac echo-Doppler, 343
Caruncular lesion, 219, 219f
    elevated round, 232
    pigmented, 220–221, 221f
Caruncular nevus, 219f–220f, 220
Cataract
    anterior polar, 391f–392f, 392
    hypermature, 387f–388f, 388
    posterior subcapsular, 385f–386f, 386
Cataract surgery, 191, 191f, 313, 345, 361
    complications of, 383
Cataractous lens, 388f
Cavernous hemangioma
    of eyelid, 69f–70f, 70, 79f–80f, 80
    of face, 79f–80f, 80
    of orbit, 91f–92f, 92
CD3 staining, in dacryoadenitis, 86
CD20 staining, in dacryoadenitis, 86
Cells, rounded-to-polygonal-shaped, with abundant clear cytoplasm, 310f
Central corneal thinning, 186
Central retinal artery occlusion (CRAO), 325f–326f, 326
Central retinal vein occlusion, 323f–324f, 324
Chalazion, 53f–54f, 54
Chemical burn, 205, 205f
Chorioretinal scarring, 352
Chorioretinitis, *Toxoplasma*, 351f–352f, 352
Choroidal hemangioma, 277f–278f, 278
Choroidal inflammation, 380f
Choroidal mass, 305, 309, 309f
Choroidal melanoma
    after plaque therapy, 303f–304f, 304
    epithelioid type, 293f–294f, 294
Choroidal nevus, 279f–280f, 280

403